Hypermobility Syndrome

For Butterworth Heinemann:

Commissioning Editor: Heidi Allen
Development Editor: Robert Edwards
Project Manager: Pat Miller
Design direction: George Ajayi

Hypermobility Syndrome

Recognition and Management for Physiotherapists

Edited by

Rosemary Keer MSc MCSP MACP SRP
Chartered Physiotherapist, Harley Street, London, UK

Rodney Grahame CBE MD FRCP FACP
Consultant Rheumatologist, Hypermobility Clinic, Centre for Rheumatology,
University College London Hospitals, London, UK

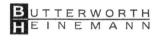

BUTTERWORTH
HEINEMANN

EDINBURGH LONDON NEW YORK OXFORD PHILADELPHIA ST LOUIS SYDNEY TORONTO 2003

BUTTERWORTH HEINEMANN
An imprint of Elsevier Limited

First published 2003
    Reprinted 2004, 2006, 2007, 2008

ISBN 978 0 7506 5390 9

British Library Cataloguing in Publication Data
A catalogue record for this book is available from the British Library

Library of Congress Cataloguing in Publication Data
A catalogue record for this book is available from the Library of
Congress

Notice
Medical knowledge is constantly changing. Standard safety
precautions must be followed, but as new research and clinical
experience broaden our knowledge, changes in treatment and drug
therapy may become necessary r appropriate. Readers are advised to
check the most current product information provided by the
manufacturer of each drug to be administered to verify the
recommended dose, the method and duration of administration, and
contraindications. It is the responsibility of the practitioner, relying on
experience and knowledge of the patient, to determine dosages and
the best treatment for each individual patient. Neither the Publisher
nor the editors assume any liability for any injury and/or damage to
persons or property arising from this publication.

ELSEVIER your source for books,
journals and multimedia
in the health sciences
www.elsevierhealth.com

Working together to grow
libraries in developing countries
www.elsevier.com | www.bookaid.org | www.sabre.org
ELSEVIER   BOOK AID   Sabre Foundation
International

The
publisher's
policy is to use
**paper manufactured
from sustainable forests**

Reproduction of Twisted Legs' sculpture on cover, courtesy of
Caroline Stacey and the Royal Society of British Sculptors

Transferred to digital print 2009

Printed and bound in Great Britain by
CPI Antony Rowe, Chippenham and Eastbourne

Contents

Contributors

Anna Edwards-Fowler BSc MCSP MACP
Chartered Physiotherapist, Central London
Physiotherapy Clinic, Harley Street, London, UK

Sarah Gurley-Green MA
Writer and Former Chairperson of the
Hypermobility Syndrome Association (HMSA),
c/o Hypermobility Clinic, Centre for
Rheumatology, University College London
Hospitals, London, UK

Vicki Harding MCSP SRP
Research and Superintendent Physiotherapist,
INPUT, St Thomas' Hospital, London, UK

Susan Maillard MCSP SRP
Chartered Physiotherapist, Paediatric
Rheumatology Unit, Great Ormond Street
Hospital, London, UK

Jean Mangharam BSc(Physio)(Hons)
MSc(Ergo / Occ Safety)
Consultant Ergonomist, Ellergo, O'Connor,
Western Australia, Australia

Elizabeth Mansi MB BS
Medical Practitioner, c/o Central London
Physiotherapy Clinic, Harley Street, London, UK

Alison Middleditch MCSP SRP
Chartered Physiotherapist, Surrey
Physiotherapy Clinic, Coulsdon, Surrey, UK

Kevin J. Murray MB BS FRACP
Consultant Paediatric Rheumatologist, Princess
Margaret Hospital for Children, Perth, Western
Australia, Australia

Jane Simmonds BPE BAppSc PGD Man Ther
Senior Lecturer in Sports Rehabilitation,
Middlesex University, Enfield, UK, and
Co-ordinator MSc Sports Physiotherapy,
University College London, London, UK

Foreword

For many years physiotherapists recognized hypermobility only as a description of an increased joint mobility above the expected norm: few recognized it as a pain syndrome. I first came upon these patients while still a novice physiotherapist. To me they were pleasant young women (I have seldom seen the same symptoms in men) whose bitter complaint of pain was not supported by the way they moved or by comparable joint signs. What is more, their symptoms were very slow to resolve. In those days, the allotted time for treatment was six to ten treatments, at which point if the patients were not better they were discharged, so most of these people were considered failures.

I had the feeling that among my colleagues these people were considered 'neurotic', and they did indeed often behave in a desperate manner. I have since come to believe that when nobody could offer them an explanation for their pain or help to relieve their symptoms they complained louder and longer in a desperate attempt to be understood – much as we are all tempted to shout when speaking to somebody who does not understand our language. It does not help, but we try it anyway.

When I qualified more than 40 years ago, I had few skills to help musculoskeletal pain, and these patients stimulated me to acquire the new techniques that were emerging at that time. When I joined the staff of Guy's Hospital in 1978, I met Professor (then Dr) Rodney Grahame, who taught me about Joint Hypermobility Syndrome (JHS). Now I had a diagnosis for my bewildering patients, but treatment was another matter. By now, I had become a member of the Manipulation Association of Chartered Physiotherapists (MACP), but even these skills were not the whole solution. In patients there appeared to be little cause and effect between their pain and activity, they had no painful range for me to improve, and it was very easy to make their symptoms worse. A survey of 100 of Professor Grahame's patients, asking them what treatment had been effective, seemed to indicate that nothing much had.

One person did give me significant help in developing a treatment regimen. She was a young doctor at Guy's and was hypermobile herself. She very quickly understood my line of questioning, and between the two of us we were able to regulate the techniques, grades and timing of mobilization that most helped her pain. As day-to-day difficulties in her life arose we looked together for practical solutions to the problems, and her medical background helped me to understand other aspects of JHS.

I am sure that other physiotherapists have trodden a similar path and will have other things to add. I know that my approach altered over the years. For others this book may be an 'Ah ha!' moment that will inspire them to persevere with a challenging but very rewarding group of patients.

Recently, interest and understanding in this subject is increasing. An informal group of therapists and doctors has been set up to exchange ideas. The many new developments in exercise regimens have improved the help we are able to give these people, and now here is a book devoted to the subject just for physiotherapists.

Anna Edwards-Fowler

Preface

People who are endowed with increased ranges of joint movement are said to be hypermobile. It is becoming clear that hypermobility is more than the curiosity it was once considered to be. There is a growing appreciation that hypermobility is more than a circus act (Grahame 2000), and that the joint hypermobility syndrome is a condition that needs to be taken seriously by all clinicians (Grahame 2001). It is becoming increasingly important in clinical practice, and in particular in physiotherapy practice, and the reason for this is that physiotherapy forms the mainstay of treatment, yet the majority of physiotherapists shy away from treating such patients because, as they report, they are at a loss to know how to treat them. It is for these colleagues that the idea for this book was conceived. It all started with a series of 1-day courses for physiotherapists interested to learn more about hypermobility and joint hypermobility syndrome (JHS), its basis, its recognition and its treatment. So far there have been courses in London, Glasgow, Bexhill-on-Sea and Norwich. Each course was oversubscribed and deemed to have been highly successful. To spread the word to a wider audience we hit on the notion of enticing the course lecturers to contribute their coursework to a book. What follows is in effect 'the book of the course'. The content is based on literature to be found in the medical and physiotherapy press, but also on the clinical experience of the authors, all of whom are involved in managing patients with JHS. Our publishers, Butterworth Heinemann, were quick to support the idea and have given us every encouragement in producing it. Our aim was to reach a much greater number of physiotherapists, both in the UK and overseas, than could ever have attended our courses. There is still much to be learnt about this condition and it is hoped that this book will stimulate interest, debate and further research.

London 2003

Rosemary Keer
Rodney Grahame

REFERENCES

Grahame, R. 2000, Hypermobility – not a circus act. [Review] [13 refs], *International Journal of Clinical Practice*, Vol. 54, No. 5, pp. 314–15.

Grahame, R. 2001, Time to take hypermobility seriously (in adults and children). [letter; comment]. [Review] [25 refs], *Rheumatology*, Vol. 40, No. 5, pp. 485–7.

1

Hypermobility and hypermobility syndrome

Rodney Grahame

Aims

This chapter aims to introduce the reader to the scientific basis of hypermobility and hypermobility syndrome, its recognition, its nomenclature, epidemiology, its clinical features and the pathogenesis of common complications, including osteoarthritis, chronic pain and recently described neurophysiological disturbances, including impairment of joint proprioception and dysautonomia, its association with certain psychiatric states and its prognosis.

INTRODUCTION

This chapter will show that inherent joint laxity is an important cause of morbidity in affected individuals. Patients thus afflicted represent a significant proportion of those seeking help for musculoskeletal symptoms from primary care physicians, rheumatologists, orthopaedic surgeons, physiotherapists and other health professionals.

It is becoming increasingly apparent to physiotherapists and other clinicians that joint hypermobility is an important entity within musculoskeletal medicine, one which hitherto has received only scant attention. There are two aspects that follow from this realization: first, that hypermobility is being frequently over-looked, disregarded or discounted; and secondly, that current approaches to treatment are often disappointingly ineffective or even detrimental. This chapter will concentrate on the recognition of hypermobility, Chapter 2 will attempt to place the hypermobility syndrome within the general context of disordered connective tissue, and

Chapter 3 will deal in general terms with the management of clinical problems that may arise.

Hypermobile joints are, by definition, those displaying a range of movement that is considered excessive taking into consideration the age, gender and ethnic background of the individual. It is important to consider these variables, as in healthy individuals joint mobility declines with age, is greater in females than in males, and varies between ethnic groups, being greatest in populations of Asian origin and least in those of European descent (Beighton et al. 1999).

THE ORIGINS OF HYPERMOBILITY

Hypermobility is the result of ligamentous laxity, which is inherent in a person's make-up and determined by their fibrous protein genes. Of particular importance in this respect are the genes that encode for collagen(s), elastin(s), fibrillin(s) and tenascin(s). Variations or mutations in such genes can give rise to the heritable disorders of connective tissue to be considered in more detail in Chapter 2.

Hypermobility may also be acquired, in the sense that joint range can also be increased, albeit with difficulty, into the hypermobile range by the sheer hard work of training. Those ballet dancers who are not endowed with inherent laxity of ligaments need to acquire hypermobility in certain joints in order to perform their art. Once they have achieved this, their basically *normal* tissues protect them against injury. Generalized joint laxity may follow in the wake of irreversible changes that occur in connective tissues in certain acquired diseases, including acromegaly, hyperparathyroidism, chronic alcoholism, systemic lupus erythematosus (SLE) and rheumatic fever (Beighton et al. 1999).

HOW TO RECOGNIZE HYPERMOBILITY

Hypermobility is easy to spot if you look for it. It is equally easy to miss it if you do not. The reality is that instruction in the techniques for recognizing hypermobility is often omitted from student clinical curricula. For example, only one major international rheumatology textbook provides such instruction (Grahame 1998). Until it becomes fully established as a routine part of every clinical examination, hypermobility will continue to be overlooked and its significance missed. As a result, patients will continue to be deprived of the relief they are seeking (Gurley-Green 2001).

A popular screening technique for hypermobility is the nine-point scale known as the Beighton score (Beighton et al. 1973). This requires the performance of five manoeuvres (four passive, one active; four bilateral, one unilateral), which are listed in Box 1.1 and demonstrated in Figure 1.1. The Beighton score was originally introduced for epidemiological studies involving the recognition of hypermobility in populations. For this task it was well suited, being easy and quick to perform even in large numbers of people. Unfortunately, it was seized on by clinicians for use as a diagnostic test for hypermobility, and hence for hypermobility syndrome (see below), a role for which it is not particularly well suited for two principal reasons. First, it samples only a small number of joints for examination, so that hypermobile joints outside this selected group will inevitably and invariably tend to be overlooked. This becomes particularly

Box 1.1 Nine-point Beighton hypermobility score		
The ability to:	Right	Left
1. Passively dorsiflex the fifth metacarpophalangeal joint to $\geqslant 90°$	1	1
2. Passively appose the thumb to the volar aspect of the forearm	1	1
3. Passively hyperextend the elbow to $\geqslant 10°$	1	1
4. Passively hyperextend the knee to $\geqslant 10°$	1	1
5. Actively place hands flat on the floor without bending the knees	1	
Total		9

One point may be gained for each side for manoeuvres 1–4 so that the hypermobility score will have a maximum of nine points if all are positive.

important once it is appreciated that joint hypermobility occurs more frequently in pauciarticular (one to four joints) distribution than in polyarticular (five or more joints) distribution (Larsson et al. 1987, 1993a, Van Dongen et al. 1999). Secondly, it is an 'all-or-none' test. It gives no indication of the degree of hypermobility, merely an expression of the widespread nature (or otherwise) of its distribution. To a certain extent the latter failing can be overcome by adopting the semiquantitative modification of the Beighton score

known as the Contompasis score (McNerney 1979), although it is more time-consuming to perform. In effect, it gives a much more refined grading by allowing between two and six (eight in the case of the forward flexion test) points for each of the nine Beighton ones, giving a possible total score of between two and 54 points. In so doing it also provides a means of measuring joint range from the hypomobility end of the spectrum, through the normal range and into the hypermobile range. In addition (being himself a podiatrist),

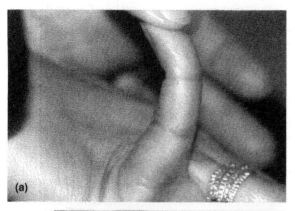

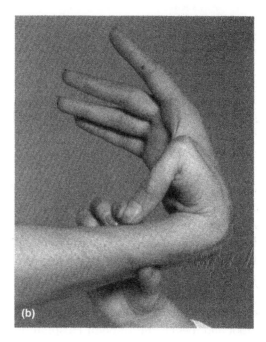

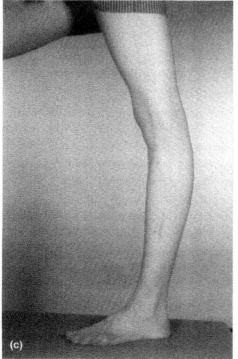

Figure 1.1a–c The nine-point Beighton score for identifying hypermobility. Shown are: (a) hyperextension of the 5th metacarpophalangeal joint to 90°; (b) apposition of the thumb to the volar aspect of the forearm; (c) hyperextension of the knee to ⩾10°

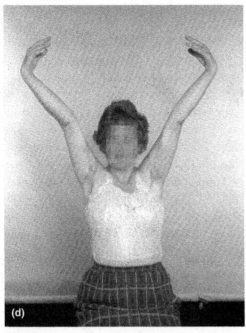 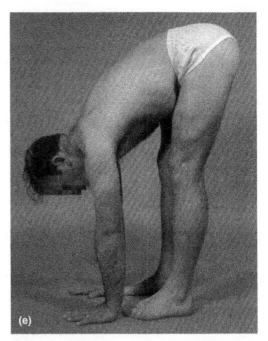

Figure 1.1d, e (d) hyperextension of the elbow to ⩾10°; (e) ability to place the hands flat on the floor with spine flexed and knees extended

Contompasis introduces a sixth test, a test of hindfoot eversion with a range of between two and seven points. If the foot eversion test is included, the maximal range extends from two to 70 points. The complete Contompasis scoring system is shown in Box 1.2.

An alternative scale that offers a wider view of joint laxity (including the shoulder, hip, patella ankle, foot and toes) is the 10-point Hospital del Mar (Barcelona) criteria (Bulbena et al. 1992).

Clearly, the search for hypermobile joints in the clinical setting should look beyond the few that constitute the Beighton score. There are several other joint areas that can easily yield useful evidence. Some of these have been incorporated into the Barcelona scale. A selection favoured by the author are listed in Box 1.3 and shown in Figure 1.2.

There is no doubt that hypermobility can prove an asset, particularly to those who engage in the performing arts, such as dancers, musicians, gymnasts, acrobats and contortionists, where exceptional ranges of movement are required (Larsson et al. 1993b, Grahame 1993). There is evidence that hypermobility may act as a positive selection factor for entry into ballet school (Grahame and Jenkins 1972, McCormack 2002, personal communication).

HYPERMOBILITY OR HYPERMOBILITY SYNDROME?

The acknowledgement within medical circles that joint hypermobility can be responsible for the production of distressing and disabling symptoms has been slow in coming. There are still many rheumatologists who remain sceptical about this (Grahame 2001). The credit for being the first to suggest such a link goes to Kirk, Ansell and Bywaters, who in 1967 coined the term 'hypermobility syndrome' (HMS) to describe the occurrence of musculoskeletal symptoms in 'otherwise healthy individuals', in other words, in the absence of other defined rheumatic diseases (Kirk et al. 1967) (Fig. 1.3). Other authors have subsequently suggested minor modifications to the name, namely 'joint hypermobility syndrome'

Box 1.2 The Contompasis semi-quantitative scoring system for hypermobility

1. Passive apposition of the thumb to the flexor aspects of the forearm ('thumb to wrist test'). Points are allocated according to the extent to which the thumb meets or passes the forearm as follows:

Thumb and forearm not touching and separated by between 30° and 75°	2
Thumb touches the forearm	4
Thumb digs into the forearm easily	5
Thumb can be pushed beyond the axis of the forearm	6

2. Passive dorsiflexion of the fifth metacarpophalangeal joint. The angle measured is the long axis of the forearm with the long axis of the fifth digit:

Hyperextension between 30° and 85°	2
Hyperextension of 90°–100°	4
Hyperextension of 100°–120°	5
Hyperextension >120°	6

3. Passive hyperextension of the elbow. The angle measured is the long axis of the forearm with the long axis of the upper arm:

Hyperextension between 0° and 5°	2
Hyperextension between 10° and 15°	4
Hyperextension between 16° and 20°	5
Hyperextension >20°	6

4. Passive hyperextension of the knee:

Hyperextension of 0°–5°	2
Hyperextension of 10°–15°	4
Hyperextension of 16°–20°	5
Hyperextension >20°	6

5. Forward flexion of the spine, attempting to place the hands flat on the floor in front of the feet (which are together) without bending the knees:

No contact with the ground	2
Fingertips touch the ground	4
Fingers touch the ground	5
Palms can be placed flat on the ground	6
Wrists can be placed on the ground	7
Forearm reaches the ground	8

6. Foot flexibility test (ankle dorsiflexion and calcaneal stance position). The degree of eversion of the calcaneus is recorded:

0°–2° of eversion	2
3°–5° of eversion	4
6°–10° of eversion	5
11°–15° of eversion	6
>15° of eversion	7

It will be noted that five of these six movements replicate Beighton et al.'s (1973) modification of the Carter and Wilkinson (1964) scoring system, but by allocating a greater range of points to the degree of hyperlaxity achieved (2–56, foot test excluded; 2–70, foot test included)

Box 1.3 Looking for hypermobility – potentially fruitful areas

- Hands and fingers outstretched (Fig. 1.2b)
- Wrist flexion and extension
- Lateral rotation of the shoulder (90° or more)
- Cervical spine (rotation to left or right to 90° or more; lateral flexion to left or right >60°).
- Temporomandibular joint (ability to insert four fingers vertically placed one above the other into mouth).
- Dorsal spine (ability to rotate passively to 90°)
- Hip rotation (medial + lateral rotation = 150°)
- Ankle (flexion + extension = 90° or more)
- Passive hyperextension of the MTP joint of big toe 90° or more (Fig. 1.2e)

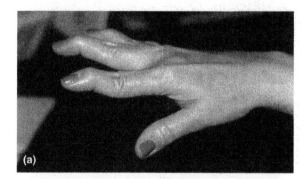

(a)

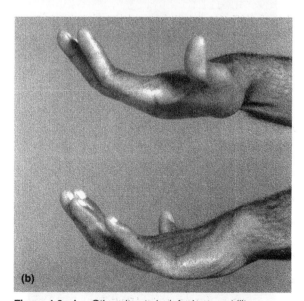

(b)

Figure 1.2a, b Other sites to look for hypermobility. (a) Hand fully extended mimicking the 'swan-neck deformity'. (b) Fully extended hand demonstrating the upward curve signifying hyperextension at the metacarpophalangeal, proximal and distal interphalangeal joints

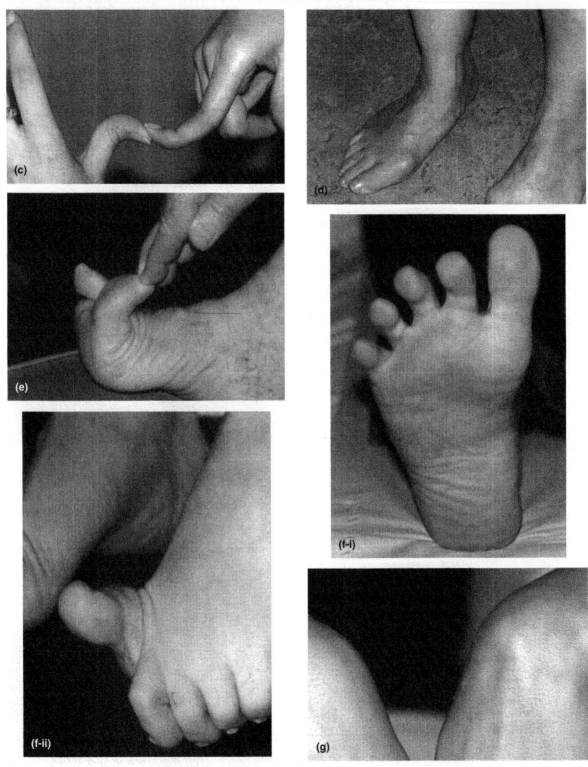

Figure 1.2c–g (c) The hyperextended interphalangeal joint of the thumb and metacarpophalangeal, proximal and distal interphalangeal joints of the index finger. (d) The foot, which becomes flat on weight bearing. (e) Passive hyperextension of the first metatarsophalangeal joint to 90°. (f) Active hypermobility of the foot – active abduction of the toes. (g) Active hyperflexion of the wrist showing a subluxing carpal bone on the left with a normal appearance on the right

(JHS) and 'benign joint hypermobility syndrome' (BJHS), but all three terms are used synonymously. The adjective 'benign' was introduced in the 1990s when it became clear that life-threatening complications did not form part of the clinical picture (Mishra et al. 1996). It subsequently also became clear that many patients suffer from a miserable existence arising from pain and other symptoms (to be documented below), so that the epithet 'benign' has become objectionable to many patients, and therefore in deference to them it should be dropped. For this reason the term 'joint hypermobility syndrome' (JHS) will be used exclusively through-out this book. As will be discussed below, JHS and Ehlers–Danlos syndrome – hypermobility type, formerly referred to as Ehlers–Danlos type 3 (EDS III) – are considered by many authorities to be one and the same.

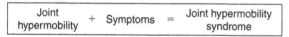

Figure 1.3 People with hypermobile joints are simply hypermobile people. Hypermobile people with musculoskeletal symptoms may be deemed to have the hypermobility syndrome, provided those symptoms are derived from the hypermobility and not from some other cause

What is the nature of hypermobility and the joint hypermobility syndrome?

There are two schools of thought. Some rheumatologists see hypermobility as a physiological variation in the range of joint movement, the uppermost range of a normal distribution within a given population. They acknowledge that such individuals may experience pain in their joints after exercise, but see this as a minor problem which is unlikely to impair that person's quality of life. In essence, it is seen as a physiological problem rather than a pathological one. Furthermore, they do not see JHS as a condition to be taken seriously (Grahame 2001). This was demonstrated in a recent survey of 319 UK-based British consultant rheumatologist members of the British Society

for Rheumatology (Grahame and Bird 2001), 72% of whom felt that it made only a minimal contribution to the overall burden of rheumatic disease morbidity. Although referral for physiotherapy was widely practised, 55% of respondents felt that it was not very effective or useless. Of those who advocated reassurance only as an appropriate method of management (88% of the total sample), 56% thought that it was an effective treatment, a view likely to be strongly disputed by the patients themselves (Gurley-Green 2001).

The other view (shared by this author) is that JHS is in effect a pathological entity, a member of the family of conditions called the heritable disorders of connective tissue (HDCTs) (Grahame 1999) (see Chapter 2). This is based on the finding of evidence of skin involvement with increased stretchiness (hyperextensibility), thin crinkly scars and striae atrophicae, which develop during adolescence.

HOW COMMON IS HYPERMOBILITY IN THE POPULATION?

There is a paucity of good epidemiological data on hypermobility. Surveys have shown wide variation in prevalence between the different groups or populations studied. There is a general consensus that hypermobility declines during childhood and adult life (Silverman et al. 1975), is more common in females than in males, and varies among ethnic groups, so that it is greatest in those of Asian origin, followed by those of African descent and least of all in Europeans (Beighton et al. 1999). The highest prevalences in groups studied to date were those found in Iraqi students (Al-Rawi et al. 1985) and the Noruba tribe in Nigeria, among 240 of whom aged 6–66 years it was found that 43% (M 35%; F 57%) scored >3/9 on the Beighton scale (Birrell et al. 1994). What is even less certain is how common JHS is in the general population. One of the difficulties in ascertaining the true prevalence of JHS in the community hitherto has been the lack of a reliable definition to use in population surveys. Now that the 1998 Brighton Criteria have been published the situation is ripe for change (Grahame et al. 2000) (see Box 1.4).

THE CLINICAL FEATURES OF JHS

The clinical features of JHS are very variable in terms of their nature, severity and occurrence. Pain is the overriding symptom and can arise from several mechanisms.

1. First and foremost is the predisposition to the effects of trauma (of either the acute or the more chronic overuse varieties) that results from having fragile connective tissues. Because collagen and other matrix fibrous proteins constitute the infrastructure of so many tissues throughout the body, the whole panoply of soft tissues is susceptible. These are summarized in Table 1.1. The most commonly affected are ligament, joint capsule, muscle, tendon, tendon–osseous junction, skin and bone. Physiotherapists treating such lesions should bear in mind that in JHS patients healing is likely to be slow and hence rehabilitation prolonged. All areas that are 'weak spots' in everyone, such as the tendo Achilles, patellofemoral joint, rotator cuff, carpal tunnel, lateral and medial epicondyles, cervical and lumbar spines (to mention a few), will be doubly susceptible in JHS subjects. Those in physically demanding occupations or those taking part in vigorous leisure activities or any unaccustomed physical activity will be at greatest risk. Multiple simultaneous painful

lesions are not uncommon. In one study the mean number of painful sites among a group of 51 patients was 8.1 (Sacheti et al. 1997).

2. JHS has long since been suspected of being a risk factor for the development of premature osteoarthritis (OA). The precise relative risk has not been determined, but a clear statistical association has been established in two Icelandic studies between hypermobility and generalized osteoarthritis of the hand (GOA) (Jonsson and Valtysdottir 1995), and more specifically to the thumb base (first carpometacarpal) joint (Jonsson et al. 1996). In the latter study thumb base OA was more common, advanced and disabling in hypermobile patients than in matched controls. In hypermobile patients the OA was more severe at the thumb base and less so in the interphalangeal joints, whereas in the controls the contrary was the case. The spinal equivalent of OA, spondylosis, whether in the cervical, thoracic or lumbar region, is seen as a common accompaniment to JHS in clinical practice, not infrequently as a presenting symptom.

3. Fibromyalgia syndrome (FMS) is frequently diagnosed in hypermobile subjects and its relationship to JHS is uncertain and controversial. The diagnosis of FMS is generally based on the 1990 American College of Rheumatology criteria (Wolfe et al. 1990). These are based on a history of widespread chronic pain and the finding of 'tender points' (TP) at specific designated sites. There is clear evidence of a statistical association between hypermobility and FMS in both adults and children (Acasuso-Diaz

Table 1.1 Joint hypermobility syndrome – clinical features

Joint	Soft tissue	Spine	Extra-articular
Hip dysplasia Late walking	Ligament/muscle/meniscus tear	'Loose back' syndrome	Stretchy skin, thin scars
'Growing pains'	Epicondylitis	Disc prolapse	Hernia
Arthralgia/myalgia	Tendonitis/capsulitis	Pars defects	Varicose veins, fractures
Dislocation/subluxation	Tenosynovitis, entrapment neuropathy	Spondylolysis/listhesis	Uterine/rectal
Joint synovitis	Fibromyalgia	Spinal anomalies	Prolapse
Chondromalacia patellae	Baker's cyst	Spinal stenosis	Chronic pain syndrome
Osteoarthritis	Fibromyalgia	SI joint instability	Depression/anxiety

and Collantes-Esteves 1998, Gedalia et al. 2000). However, Karaaslan et al. (2000) found evidence that JHS patients frequently manifested TP that did not conform with the ACR criteria, and thus were at risk of being misdiagnosed as having FMS. Fibromyalgia is no longer looked upon by most rheumatologists as a specific pathological entity as it once was, but more of a non-specific 'cry for help' from someone in a distressed state.

OTHER PHYSIOLOGICAL AND PSYCHOLOGICAL ABNORMALITIES

It has come to light over the past decade that patients with JHS are susceptible to a complex array of neurophysiological defects and psychiatric ailments, which explains why so many of them complain of symptoms that relate to organs and systems remote from the musculoskeletal system. Hitherto, these have been unexplained and therefore largely discounted, and in many cases simply not believed. These comprise:

- Impairment of joint proprioceptive acuity, demonstrated in the proximal interphalangeal joint and knee (Mallik et al. 1994, Hall et al. 1995). It should be pointed out that the degree of impairment is not detectable on clinical examination and only on using sophisticated equipment. Nevertheless, it could have an adverse effect by compromising balance and coordination.
- Lack of efficacy of local anaesthetics topically applied or given by injection (Arendt-Nielsen et al. 1990). The mechanism is unknown. However, it can cause consternation and distress to the unwary in the dental surgery, during childbirth (when epidural anaesthesia is used) or during minor surgery.
- Pain enhancement, leading to the development of a full chronic pain syndrome, an all-too-frequent complication of JHS, where pain, both acute and chronic, becomes the dominant factor

in people's daily life and is allowed to pursue its inexorable course in the absence of effective treatment. Chronic pain and its management is a recurring theme in later chapters of this book.

- From the early 1990s a group of researchers in Spain (Bulbena et al. 1993) have drawn attention to a significant association between hypermobility and anxiety states with panic attacks and phobic states. Panic disorder, agoraphobia and simple phobias were four times more common in hypermobile patients than in controls, whereas joint laxity was 16 times more common in patients with panic/agoraphobia than in controls (Bulbena et al. 1988, 1993). A similar association was encountered in a community setting (Martin-Santos et al. 1998). In 2001 the same group reported a genetic link between anxiety, phobia and hypermobility in the form of a chromosomal duplication on chromosome 15 (15q 24-26), which the authors proposed as a susceptibility factor for a clinical phenotype that included panic and phobic disorders and joint laxity (Gratacos 2001).
- Autonomic dysfunction has very recently been added to the spectrum of neurophysiological disorders in JHS. JHS patients not infrequently complain of symptoms such as palpitations, light-headedness, dizziness or fainting, which are similar to those experienced by people with autonomic nervous system dysfunction. In a carefully controlled study (Gazit et al. 2003) 48 female JHS patients completed a questionnaire which showed that over a range of symptoms suggestive of autonomic dysfunction, their response was strongly positive. Furthermore, in an extension to the study 27 patients and 21 controls underwent a series of tests of autonomic function, including the orthostatic test, measurement of catecholamine levels, tests of vagal and sympathetic control and cardiovascular adrenoreceptor responsiveness. There was a highly significant difference between patients and controls, with 22% and 15% of patients matching the criteria for orthostatic hypotension and postural orthostatic tachycardia

syndrome, respectively. A further 48% had an uncategorized orthostatic intolerance, compared to only 9.5% of controls. The pathogenetic basis for these striking results remains to be determined.

Thus it will be seen that the manifestations of JHS are manifold and various and the ramifications extend far from the tissue laxity notion with which it was originally associated. An A–Z compendium of 77 JHS symptoms and reported associations is appended together with references as Box 1.5.

The diagnosis of joint hypermobility syndrome is based on a typical history, a finding of consistent lesions and other clinical features (as listed in Box 1.5), together with the finding of hypermobility and/or other features of JHS. The recently published 1998 Brighton Criteria for the Benign Joint Hypermobility Syndrome is a validated set of criteria which goes far beyond the nine-point Beighton score and takes account of patients' symptoms and also other stigmata of connective tissue deficiency (Grahame et al. 2000). It is shown in Box 1.4. Although devised primarily for phenotypic recognition of JHS in research protocols, it is proving to be a useful clinical diagnostic tool. Caution is, however, advised against using it as for diagnostic purposes in too rigid a manner. It has, for example, not yet been validated for use in children below the age of 16, or for elderly people. Because the exclusion of MFS and EDS (other than EDS III) may be required, it should be used in conjunction with the Ghent criteria (De Paepe et al. 1996) for MFS and the Villefranche criteria (Beighton et al. 1998) for EDS (see Chapter 2).

PROGNOSIS

It is widely recognized that hypermobility (and any individual's hypermobility score) diminishes throughout life. From this it has tended to be assumed that the symptoms associated with hypermobility will also diminish with age. Sadly, this

---

Box 1.4   Revised diagnostic criteria for the benign joint hypermobility syndrome (BJHS) (Grahame et al. 2000)

Major criteria
1. A Beighton score of 4/9 or greater (either currently or historically)
2. Arthralgia for longer than 3 months in four or more joints.

Minor criteria
1. A Beighton score of 1, 2 or 3/9 (0, 1, 2 or 3 if aged 50+)
2. Arthralgia (≥3 months) in one to three joints or back pain (≥3 months), spondylosis, spondylolysis/spondylolisthesis
3. Dislocation/subluxation in more than one joint, or in one joint on more than one occasion
4. Soft tissue rheumatism. Three or more lesions (e.g. epicondylitis, tenosynovitis, bursitis)
5. Marfanoid habitus (tall, slim, span/height ratio > 1.03, upper:lower segment ratio less than 0.89, arachnodactyly (positive Steinberg/wrist signs)
6. Abnormal skin: striae, hyperextensibility, thin skin, papyraceous scarring
7. Eye signs: drooping eyelids or myopia or antimongoloid slant
8. Varicose veins or hernia or uterine/rectal prolapse.

BJHS is diagnosed in the presence of **two** major criteria, or **one** major and **two** minor criteria, or **four** minor criteria. **Two** minor criteria will suffice where there is an unequivocally affected first-degree relative. BJHS is excluded by presence of Marfan or Ehlers–Danlos syndromes other than the EDS hypermobility type (formerly EDS III) as defined by the Ghent (De Paepe 1996) and the Villefranche (Beighton et al. 1998) criteria, respectively. Criteria Major 1 and Minor 1 are mutually exclusive, as are Major 2 and Minor 2.

---

does not appear to be the case. Studies have shown that for many, JHS commences in childhood or adolescence and is carried forward into adult life. Rather than diminishing in severity, it appears to become more vicious and disruptive of daily life (Sacheti et al. 1997, Gurley-Green 2001). A number of factors conspire to generate the downward spiral. These include:

• the severity of the condition and frequency of 'medical events';
• lack of understanding and appropriate treatment offered by health professionals;
• conflicting demands and pressures from work and family commitments;
• lack of coping skills;
• kinesiphobia (fear of pain induced by movement), leading to disuse and deconditioning.

Clearly, for patients who enter this spiral the future is, indeed, bleak unless heroic measures are undertaken. Strategies to prevent this state of affairs or to counteract the effects are considered in Chapter 3 and subsequent chapters throughout the book. It should be emphasized that only a minority of JHS patients will suffer such severe symptoms. Milder cases predominate, especially in the earlier phases of the disorder, where symptoms are episodic rather than perennial. There does seem to be one time of life when JHS patients enjoy a respite, and that is in old age. Currently the evidence is anecdotal, but clinical experience strongly suggests that elderly hypermobile subjects are more agile and more active than their normally mobile peers. This enables them to remain more physically and thereby more mentally active. A recently published epidemiological survey carried out among 716 women in Chingford (age range 53–72, mean 61; SD 5.8) on the outskirts of London found that those with evidence of hypermobility were fitter than the rest and showed a higher bone mineral density and a lower incidence of osteoarthritis of the knee (Dolan et al. 2001). There is one aspect of the prognosis in JHS which does not appear to be in doubt: according to the available evidence, life expectancy is not diminished and the life-threatening complications that occur in other more serious heritable disorders of connective tissue (see Chapter 2), such as aortic dilatation, mercifully do not affect patients with JHS (Mishra et al. 1996).

Box 1.5   An A–Z compendium of 77 JHS symptoms and associations with references

A   Abdominal pain (Sacheti et al. 1997)
Anterior knee pain (Al-Rawi and Nessan 1997)
Anxiety (Bulbena et al. 1993)
Arthralgia (Beighton et al. 1999)
Autonomic dysfunction (Gazit 2003)
B   Back pain (Beighton et al. 1999)
Baker's cyst (Grahame 1971)
Breast implant (Lai et al. 2000)
C   Capsulitis of the shoulder (Hudson et al. 1995)
Carpal tunnel syndrome (March et al. 1988)
Cervical spondylosis (Beighton et al. 1999)
Chondromalacia patellae (Al-Rawi and Nessan 1997)
Chronic pain syndrome (Grahame 2000)
Cystocele (Norton et al. 1995)
D   Deconditioning
Depression (Lumley et al. 1994)
Disc prolapse (Morgan et al. 1996)
Dislocation (Runow 1982)
E   Entrapment neuropathy (March et al. 1988)
Epicondylitis (Hudson et al. 1995)
F   Fainting (Gazit 2003)
Fatigue (Rowe et al. 1999)
Fibromyalgia (Acasuso-Diaz and Collantes-Estevez 1998); (Gedalia et al. 2000)
Flat feet (Beighton et al. 1999)
Fractures (Grahame et al. 1981)
G   'Growing pains' (Southwood 1993)
H   Haemorrhoids (Al-Rawi 2000a, *Iraqi Postgraduate Medical Journal* (in press))
Headaches (Blau 1999)
Hernia (Wynne-Davies 1971)
Hiatus hernia (Al-Rawi 2002, personal communication)
Hip dysplasia (Dubs and Gschwend 1988)
Hypotension, orthostatic (Gazit 2003)

I   Instability (Runow 1982)
J   Joint synovitis (Beighton et al. 1999)
K   Knee pain (Al-Rawi and Nessan 1997)
Kinesiphobia (Vlaeyen and Linton 2000)
L   Late walking (Davidovitch et al. 1994)
Ligament tear (Diaz et al. 1993)
Lid laxity (Mishra et al. 1996)
Lignocaine resistance (Arendt-Nielsen 1990)
'Loose-back syndrome' (Howes et al. 1971)
M   Marfanoid habitus (Grahame et al. 1981)
Meniscus tear (Bird et al. 1980)
Mitral valve prolapse (Grahame et al. 1981; Mishra et al. 1996)
Muscle tear (Beighton et al. 1999)
Myalgia (Beighton et al. 1999)
N   Neck pain (Beighton et al. 1999)
O   Osteoarthritis (Jonsson and Valtysdottir 1995) (Jonsson et al. 1996)
P   Pain augmentation (Grahame 2000)
Panic attacks (Bulbena et al. 1988; Bulbena 1993; Martin-Santos et al. 1998)
Pars interarticularis defects (Beighton et al. 1999)
Pes planus (Beighton et al. 1999)
Phobic states (Bulbena et al. 1988; Bulbena 1993; Martin-Santos et al. 1998)
Plantar fasciitis (Beighton et al. 1999)
Premature labour (Barabas 1966)
Procidentia (Norton et al.1995)
Proprioceptive impairment (Mallik et al. 1994)
Q   Quantification of hyperlaxity (Beighton et al. 1988)
R   Rectal prolapse (Marshman 1987)
Rectocele (Norton et al. 1995)
S   Sacroiliac joint instability (Beighton et al. 1999)
Scoliosis (Grahame et al. 1981)

Box 1.5 Cont'd

Spinal anomalies (Grahame et al. 1981)
Spinal stenosis (Beighton et al. 1999)
Spondylolysis (Beighton et al. 1999)
Spondylolisthesis (Morgan et al. 1996)
Sprains (Diaz et al. 1993)
Stress incontinence (Zafirakis and Grahame 2002)
Stretchy skin (Mishra et al. 1996)
Subluxation (Beighton et al. 1999)
T Temporomandibular dysfunction
(Beighton et al. 1999)

Tendonitis (Beighton et al. 1999)
Tenosynovitis (Beighton et al. 1999)
Thin scars (Beighton et al. 1999)
U Uterine prolapse (Norton et al. 1995)
V Varicose veins (Al-Rawi et al. 1985)
W Woodwind players (Larsson et al. 1993b)
X Tenascin-X (Chapter 2) (Schalkwijk et al. 2001)
Y Young's modulus for collagen
(Beighton et al. 1999)
Z Zygapophyseal joints (Beighton et al. 1999)

REFERENCES

Acasuso-Diaz, M. and Collantes-Estevez, E. (1998) Joint hypermobility in patients with fibromyalgia syndrome. *Arthritis Care and Research*, **11**, 39–42.

Al-Rawi, Z.S., Al-Aszawi, A.J. and Al-Chalabi, T. (1985) Joint mobility amongst university students. *British Journal of Rheumatology*, **24**, 326–31.

Al-Rawi, Z. and Nessan, A.H. (1997) Joint hypermobility in patients with chondromalacia patellae. *British Journal of Rheumatology*, **36**, 1324–7.

Arendt-Nielsen, L., Kaalund, P., Bjerring, P. and Hogsaa, B. (1990) Insufficient effect of local analgesics in Ehlers–Danlos type III patients (connective tissue disorder). *Acta Anaesthesiologica Scandinavica*, **34**, 358–61.

Barabas, A.P. (1966) Ehlers–Danlos syndrome associated with prematurity, premature rupture of the membranes; possible increase in incidence. *British Medical Journal*, **2**, 682–4.

Beighton, P.H., Soskolne, L. and Solomon, C.L. (1973) Articular mobility in an African population. *Annals of the Rheumatic Diseases*, **32**, 413–17.

Beighton, P.H., De Paepe, A., Steinmann, B. et al. (1998) Ehlers–Danlos syndromes: revised nosology, Villefranche, 1997. Ehlers–Danlos National Foundation (USA) and Ehlers–Danlos Support Group (UK). *American Journal of Medical Genetics*, **77**, 31–7.

Beighton, P.H., Grahame, R. and Bird, H. (1999) *Hypermobility of Joints*, 3rd edn. Springer-Verlag.

Bird, H.A., Hudson, A., Eastmond, C.J. and Wright, V. (1980) Joint laxity and osteoarthritis: a radiological survey of female physical education specialists. *British Journal of Sports Medicine*, **14**, 179–88.

Birrell, F.N., Adebajo, A.O., Hazleman, B.L., and Silman, A.J. (1994) High prevalence of joint laxity in West Africans. *British Journal of Rheumatology*, **33**, 56–9.

Blau, J.N. (1999) Joint hypermobility and headache. [letter; comment]. *Cephalalgia*, **19**, 765–6.

Bulbena, A., Duro, J.C., Mateo, A. et al. (1988) Joint hypermobility syndrome and anxiety disorders. *Lancet*, **2**, 694.

Bulbena, A., Duro, J.C., Porta, M. et al. (1992) Clinical assessment of hypermobility of joints: assembling criteria. *Journal of Rheumatology*, **19**, 115–22.

Bulbena, A., Duro, J.C., Porta, M. et al. (1993) Anxiety disorders in the joint hypermobility syndrome. *Psychiatry Research*, **46**, 59–68.

Carter, C. and Wilkinson, J. (1964) Persistent joint laxity and congenital dislocation of the hip. *Journal of Bone Joint Surgery [Br]*, **46**, 40–5.

Davidovitch, M., Tirosh, E. and Tal, Y. (1994) The relationship between joint hypermobility and neurodevelopmental attributes in elementary school children. *Journal of Child Neurology*, **9**, 417–19.

De Paepe, A., Devereux, R.B., Dietz, H.C. et al. (1996) Revised diagnostic criteria for the Marfan syndrome. *American Journal of Medical Genetics*, **62**, 417–26.

Diaz, M.A., Estevez, E.C. and Sanchez, G.P. (1993) Joint hyperlaxity and musculoligamentous lesions: study of a population of homogeneous age, sex and physical exertion. *British Journal of Rheumatology*, **32**, 120–2.

Dolan, A.L., Hart, D.J., Doyle, D.V. et al. (2003) The relationship of joint hypermobility, bone mineral density, and osteoarthritis in the general population: the Chingford study. *Journal of Rheumatology*, **30**, 799–803.

Dubs, L. and Gschwend, N. (1988) General joint laxity. Quantification and clinical relevance. *Archives of Orthopedic and Trauma Surgery*, **107**, 65–72.

Gazit, Y., Nahir, A.M., Grahame, R. and Jacob, G. (2003) Dysautonomia in the joint hypermobility syndrome. *American Journal of Medicine*, **115**, 33–40.

Gedalia, A., Garcia, C.O., Molina, J.F. et al. (2000) Fibromyalgia syndrome: experience in a pediatric rheumatology clinic. *Clinical and Experimental Rheumatology*, **18**, 415–19.

Grahame, R. (1971) Joint hypermobility – clinical aspects. *Proceedings of the Royal Society of Medicine*, **64**, 692–4.

Grahame, R. (1993) Joint hypermobility and the performing musician [editorial; comment]. *New England Journal of Medicine*, **329**, 1120–1.

Grahame, R. (1998) Examination of the joints. In *Rheumatology*, 2nd edn. (J.H. Klippel and P.A. Dieppe, eds), pp. 1–16, Mosby.

Grahame, R. (1999) Joint hypermobility and genetic collagen disorders: are they related? *Archives of Disease in Childhood*, **80**, 188–91.

Grahame, R. (2000) Pain, distress and joint hyperlaxity. *Joint Bone Spine*, **67**, 157–63.

Grahame, R. (2001) Time to take hypermobility seriously (in adults and children). *Rheumatology*, **40**, 485–7.

Grahame, R. (2002) Comment – Ten myths about hypermobility. *Current Medical Literature – Rheumatology*, **21**, 29–32.

Grahame, R. and Bird, H.A. (2001) British consultant rheumatologists' perceptions about the hypermobility syndrome. *Rheumatology*, **40**, 559–62.

Grahame, R., Bird, H.A., Child, A. et al. (2000) The revised (Brighton 1998) criteria for the diagnosis of benign joint hypermobility syndrome (BJHS). *Journal of Rheumatology*, **27**, 1777–9.

Grahame, R., Edwards, J.C., Pitcher, D. et al. (1981) A clinical and echocardiographic study of patients with the hypermobility syndrome. *Annals of the Rheumatic Diseases*, **40**, 541–6.

Grahame, R. and Jenkins, J.M. (1972) Joint hypermobility – asset or liability? A study of joint mobility in ballet dancers. *Annals of the Rheumatic Diseases*, **31**, 2, 109–11.

Gratacos, M., Martin-Santos, N. et al. (2001) A polymorphic genomic duplication on human chromosome 15 is a susceptibility factor for panic and phobic disorders. *Cell*, **106**, 367–79.

Gurley-Green, S. (2001) Living with the hypermobility syndrome. [see comments]. *Rheumatology*, **40**, 487–9.

Hall, M.G., Ferrell, W.R., Sturrock, R.D. et al. (1995) The effect of the hypermobility syndrome on knee joint proprioception. *British Journal of Rheumatology*, **34**, 121–5.

Howes, R.J. and Isdale, I.C. (1971) The loose back: an unrecognised syndrome. *Rheumatology and Physical Medicine*, **11**, 72–7.

Hudson, N., Starr, M.R., Esdaile, J.M. and Fitzcharles, M.-A. (1995) Diagnostic associations with hypermobility in rheumatology patients. *British Journal of Rheumatology*, **34**, 1157–61.

Jonsson, H. and Valtysdottir, S.T. (1995) Hypermobility features in patients with hand osteoarthritis. *Osteoarthritis and Cartilage*, **3**, 1–5.

Jonsson, H., Valtysdottir, S.T., Kjartansson, O. and Brekkan, A. (1996) Hypermobility associated with osteoarthritis of the thumb base: a clinical and radiological subset of hand osteoarthritis. *Annals of the Rheumatic Diseases*, **55**, 540–3.

Karaaslan, Y., Haznedaroglu, S. and Ozturk, M. (2000) Joint hypermobility and primary fibromyalgia: a clinical enigma. [see comments]. *Journal of Rheumatology*, **27**, 1774–6.

Kirk, J.H., Ansell, B. and Bywaters, E.G.L. (1967) The hypermobility syndrome. *Annals of the Rheumatic Diseases*, **26**, 425.

Lai, S., Goldman, J.A., Child, A.H. et al. (2000) Fibromyalgia, hypermobility and breast implants. *Journal of Rheumatology*, **27**, 2237–41.

Larsson, L.-G., Baum, J. and Mudholkar, G.S. (1987) Hypermobility: features and differential incidence between the sexes. *Arthritis and Rheumatism*, **30**, 1426–30.

Larsson, L.-G., Baum, J., Muldolkar, G.S. and Srivastava, D.K. (1993a) Hypermobility: prevalence and features in a Swedish population. *British Journal of Rheumatology*, **32**, 116–19.

Larsson, L.-G., Baum, J., Muldolkar, G.S. and Kollia, G.D. (1993b) Benefits and disadvantages of joint hypermobility among musicians. *New England Journal of Medicine*, **329**, 1079–82.

Lumley, M.A., Jordan, M., Rubenstein, R. et al. (1994) Psychosocial functioning in the Ehlers–Danlos syndrome. *American Journal of Medical Genetics*, **53**, 149–52.

Mallik, A.K., Ferrell, W.R., McDonald, A.G. and Sturrock, R.D. (1994) Impaired proprioceptive acuity at the proximal interphalangeal joint in patients with the hypermobility syndrome. *British Journal of Rheumatology*, **33**, 631–7.

March, L.M., Francis, H. and Webb, J. (1988) Benign joint hypermobility with neuropathies: documentation and mechanism of median, sciatic, and common peroneal nerve compression. *Clinical Rheumatology*, **7**, 35–40.

Marshman, D., Percy, J., Fielding, I. and Delbridge, L. (1987) Rectal prolapse: relationship with joint mobility. *Australian and New Zealand Journal of Surgery*, **57**, 827–9.

Martin-Santos, R., Bulbena, A., Porta, M. et al. (1998) Association between joint hypermobility syndrome and panic disorder. *American Journal of Psychiatry*, **155**, 1578–83.

McNerney, J.E. and Johnston, W.B. (1979) Generalised ligament laxity, hallux abducto valgus and the first metatarsocuneiform joint. *Journal of the American Podiatric Association*, **69**, 69–82.

Mishra, M.B., Ryan, P., Atkinson, P. et al. (1996) Extra-articular features of benign joint hypermobility syndrome. *British Journal of Rheumatology*, **35**, 861–6.

Morgan, A.W., Pearson, S.B. and Bird, H.A. (1996) A controlled study of spinal laxity in subjects with joint hyperlaxity and Ehlers–Danlos syndrome. *British Journal of Rheumatology*, **36**, S136 [Abstract].

Norton, P.A., Baker, J.E., Sharp, H.C. et al. (1995) Genitourinary prolapse and joint hypermobility in women. *Obstetrics and Gynecology* **85**, 225–8.

Rowe, P.B.D., Calkins, H., Maumenee, I.H. et al. (1999) Orthostatic intolerance and chronic fatigue associated with Ehlers–Danlos syndrome. *Journal of Pediatrics*, **135**, 499.

Runow, A. (1982) The dislocating patella. Etiology and prognosis in relation to joint laxity and anatomy of patellar articulation. *Acta Orthopaedica Scandinavica*, **202** (Suppl), 1–53.

Sacheti, A., Szemere, J., Bernstein, B. et al. (1997) Chronic pain is a manifestation of the Ehlers–Danlos syndrome. *Journal of Pain and Symptom Management*, **14**, 88–93.

Schalkwijk, J., Zweers, M.C., Steijlen, P. et al. (2001) A recessive form of the Ehlers–Danlos syndrome caused by tenascin-X deficiency. [see comments]. *New England Journal of Medicine*, **345**, 1167–75.

Silverman, S., Constine, L., Harvey, W. and Grahame, R. (1975) Survey of joint mobility and in vivo skin elasticity in London schoolchildren. *Annals of the Rheumatic Diseases*, **34**, 177–80.

Southwood, T.R., and Sills, J.A. (1993) Non-arthritic locomotor disorders in childhood. *Reports on the Rheumatic Diseases Series 2 Arthritis and Rheumatism Council*, Practical problems No. 24.

Van Dongen, P.W.J., De Boer, M., Lemmens, W.A.J. and Theron, G.B. (1999) Hypermobility and peripartum pelvic pain syndrome in pregnant South African women. *European Journal of Obstetrics, Gynecology, and Reproductive Biology*, **84**, 77–82.

Vlaeyen J.W.S., Linton S.J. (2000) Fear avoidance and its consequences in chronic musculoskeletal pain: a state of the art. *Pain*, **85**, 317–332.

Wolfe, F., Smythe, H.A., Yunus, M. et al. (1990) The American College of Rheumatology 1990 criteria for the classification of fibromyalgia. Report of the Multicenter Criteria Committee. *Arthritis and Rheumatism*, **33**, 160–73.

Wynne-Davies, R. (1971) Familial joint laxity. *Proceedings of the Royal Society of Medicine*, **64**, 689–90.

Zafirakis, H. and Grahame, R. (2002) Stress incontinence and BJHS. (Unpublished work)

2

Hypermobility and the heritable disorders of connective tissue

Rodney Grahame

Aims

In this chapter joint hypermobility syndrome is seen as one of the heritable disorders of connective tissue, and its similarities to and differences from the other diseases in this category are highlighted in terms of clinical features, nosological criteria and underlying molecular genetic bases. Guidelines are also provided on when it would be desirable for a physiotherapist to refer for specialist medical advice and/or for genetic testing. This chapter will attempt to place the hypermobility syndrome within the general framework of disordered connective tissue.

THE HERITABLE DISORDERS OF CONNECTIVE TISSUE (HDCTs)

These are genetic disorders affecting the genes that encode the various connective tissue matrix proteins, such as collagen(s), elastin(s), tenascin(s) and fibrillin(s). Genetic aberrations affecting these fibrous proteins distort their biochemical structure and impair their tensile physical properties, resulting in tissue laxity, fragility and, ultimately, mechanical failure (Fig. 2.1). The family of disorders is large and includes many rare and some less rare genetic disorders. It is recommended that practising physiotherapists acquire a working knowledge of the most important conditions in this group (Box 2.1). Joint hypermobility is a feature common to all the HDCTs. A résumé of the distinctive features is provided in Tables 2.1–2.5 and Box 2.2.

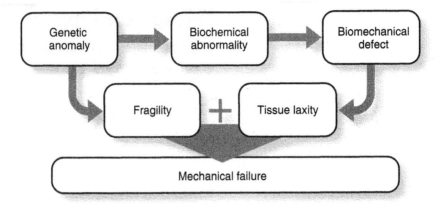

Figure 2.1 The pathophysiology that pertains in all heritable disorders of connective tissue. Genetic aberrations affecting fibrous proteins give rise to biochemical variations, then in turn to impairment of tensile strength, resulting in enhanced mobility but at a cost of increased fragility, ultimately risking mechanical tissue failure

---

Box 2.1 Common heritable disorders of connective tissue

Marfan syndrome [MFS]
Ehlers–Danlos syndrome [EDS]
Osteogenesis imperfecta [OI]
Joint hypermobility syndrome [JHS]

Table 2.1 Clinical features in Marfan syndrome (reproduced with kind permission of the editor and publishers of the Archives of Diseases of Childhood)

Site	Cardinal features	Symptoms	Effects
Joint	Hypermobility	Arthralgia	Instability
Skeleton	Marfanoid habitus	Dislocation Slender extremities Pectus deformities	Soft tissue trauma Scoliosis Arachnodactyly
Skin	Hyperextensibility	Thinning Striae atrophicae	Papyraceous scars Easy bruising
Eyes	Ectopia lentis	Visual problems	
Vascular	Aortic dilatation Mitral valve	Aneurysm Prolapse	Sub-acute bacterial endocarditis (SBE)

Table 2.2 Clinical features in the Ehlers–Danlos syndrome classic type (EDS I and II) (reproduced with kind permission of the editor and publishers of the Archives of Diseases of Childhood)

Site	Cardinal features	Symptoms	Effects
Joint	Hypermobility	Arthralgia	Instability
Skeleton	Osteoporosis	Dislocation Scoliosis Fracture	Soft tissue trauma Deformity
Skin	Hyperextensibility	Thinning Striae atrophicae Molluscoid pseudotumours	Violaceous papyraceous scars Bruising and haematomata Subcutaneous spheroids
Eyes	–	–	–
Vascular	Mitral valve Intracranial (EDS IV)	Prolapse Aneurysm	SBE Subarachnoid haemorrhage
Muscle	Laxity	Hernia Intestinal/bladder diverticulae	Rectal/uterine prolapse Neuromyopathy

Table 2.3 Clinical features in osteogenesis imperfecta (reproduced with kind permission of the editor and publishers of the Archives of Diseases of Childhood)

Site	Cardinal features	Symptoms	Effects
Joint	Hypermobility	Arthralgia	Instability
Skeleton	Osteoporosis	Dislocation Fracture	Soft tissue trauma Deformity
Skin	Hyperextensibility	Thinning Striae atrophicae	Papyraceous scars Easy bruising
Eyes	Blue sclera		
Vascular	Mitral valve	Prolapse	SBE

Table 2.4 Clinical features in the benign joint hypermobility syndrome/EDS III (reproduced with kind permission of the editor and publishers of the Archives of Diseases of Childhood)

Site	Cardinal features	Symptoms	Effects
Joint	Hypermobility	Arthralgia	Instability
Skeleton	Marfanoid habitus Osteoporosis (low BMD)	Dislocation Slender extremities Pectus deformities Fracture	Soft tissue trauma Scoliosis Arachnodactyly Deformity
Skin	Hyperextensibility	Thinning Striae atrophicae	Papyraceous scars Easy bruising
Eyes	Lid laxity Blue sclera (occasionally)		
Vascular	Varicose veins		
Muscle	Laxity	Hernia	Rectal/uterine prolapse

Table 2.5 Classification of Ehlers–Danlos syndromes (Villefranche Nosology 1997)

New	Former	OMIM	Inheritance
Classical type	Gravis EDS 1	130000	AD
	Mitis EDS II	130010	AD
Hypermobility	H/mobile EDS III	130020	AD
Vascular	Ecchymotic EDS IV	130050 (225350) (225360)	AD
Kyphoscoliosis	Ocular-Scoliotic (EDS VI)	(225400) (229200)	AR
Arthrochalasia	Arthrochalasis multiplex congenita (EDS VIIA and VIIB)	130060	
Dermatosparaxis type	EDS type VIIC	225410	AR
Other forms: X-linked EDS	(EDS type V)	305200	XL
Periodontitis type EDS VIII		130080	AD
Fibronectin-deficient EDS	(EDS type X)	225310	?
Familial h/mob syndrome	(EDS type XI)	147900	AD
Progeroid EDS		130070	?
Unspecified forms		–	

The 'Villefranche Nosology' (Beighton et al. 1998) replaced its predecessor, the 'Berlin Nosology' (Beighton et al. 1988) and, in so doing, simplified the classification of EDS, replacing the earlier numeral system with appropriate descriptive terms. (Types I and II were amalgamated to form the classic type, type III became the hypermobility type and type IV the vascular type.) The so-called familial articular hypermobility syndrome (FAHS), which previously carried the designation EDS type XI, is the one that bears the closest relation to JHS. However, it excludes skin hyperextensibility, which therefore invalidates it as a description of JHS (see Chapter 1). The numbers given refer to the OMIM classification (Online Mendelian Inheritance in Man National Center for Biotechnology Information, website http://www.ncbi.nlm.nih.gov/Omim/searchomim.html). AD, autosomal dominant pattern of inheritance; AR, autosomal recessive pattern of inheritance. *American Journal of Medical Genetics* 1998, **77**, 31–37.

Box 2.2 Revised diagnostic criteria for Marfan syndrome: the 1996 Ghent Criteria (after De Paepe et al. 1996)

Major criteria	**Minor criteria**
Skeletal – see below	Fat cornea
Ectopia lentis	Mitral valve prolapse
Dilated aorta	Pneumothorax
Dissection	Striae
Dural ectasia	
First-degree relative	
FBN1 mutation	

Skeletal criteria: the presence of four out of 12 of the following constitutes

Major criteria	**Minor criteria**
Pectus carinatum	Moderate pectus
Pectus excavatum	excavatum
requiring surgery	Joint hypermobility
Reduced upper:lower	High arched palate with
segment ratio	teeth crowding
Span:height > 1.05	Facial appearance
Positive wrist and thumb	(dolichocephaly, malar
(Steinberg) test	hypoplasia, enophthalmos,
Scoliosis > 20° or	downslanting
spondylolisthesis	palpebral fissures)
Reduced elbow extension	retrognathia
to less than 170°	
Medial displacement of	
medial malleolus to produce	
pes planus	
Protrusio acetabulae of any	
degree (ascertained on	
radiographs)	

Requirements for diagnosis of the Marfan syndrome:

For index case: Major criteria in ≥ two organ systems and involvement of a third

For relative of an index case: one major criterion + involvement of a second organ system.

THE GENETICS OF THE HDCTs

Most of the HDCTs that are commonly encountered in clinical practice (and which are discussed in this chapter) are inherited in an autosomal dominant fashion. This has practical implications for hypermobile patients who are entertaining the possibility of raising a family. Where one of the parents carries the aberrant gene there is a 50% chance, in theory, that an individual offspring will inherit the gene. In the (unlikely) event that both parents carry the mutation the odds – again in theory – increase to 100%! It should be remembered that both the manifestations and the occurrence of symptoms vary considerably

among people with the same genetic disorder, even between members of the same family, and so it is important to point out to intending parents that the occurrence and pattern of symptoms (including their nature, frequency or severity) will not necessarily be replicated in their offspring.

The most important HDCTs (from the point of view of the physiotherapist) are Marfan syndrome, Ehlers–Danlos syndrome, osteogenesis imperfecta and joint hypermobility syndrome (JHS).

Marfan syndrome (MFS)

In 1896 Antonin Marfan, an eminent Parisian physician, later to become the first French professor of paediatrics, presented a 5-year-old girl, known as Gabrielle P., with a distinctive body shape to a meeting of doctors in Paris. The now well-known and recognizable constellation of features (tall slender body with long extremities (arms, legs, hands, feet, fingers and toes), elongated head, scoliosis, pectus excavatum or carinatum, high arched palate) has universally become known as the marfanoid habitus. The characteristic body measurements and other features of the marfanoid habitus are shown in Figures 2.2 and 2.3 and Box 2.3. Over the past 100 years it has become evident that MFS can affect the eyes (causing myopia), as well as dislocation of the ocular lens (ectopia lentis) and the heart, causing mitral valve prolapse and/or aneurysm of the aorta. The cause of MFS has now been traced to one of a number of mutations of the fibrillin-1 (*FBN1*) gene. A set of MFS criteria appeared in the 1996 Berlin Nosology (Beighton 1988). These were revised and updated and subsequently published as the Ghent criteria (De Paepe et al. 1996) in the light of new knowledge, including that obtained from molecular genetic research. For the first time the notion of major and minor criteria was introduced into the classification criteria, as shown in Box 2.2.

Aortic aneurysm in MFS is a life-threatening complication because of the potential risk of aortic dissection and/or rupture. Barely three

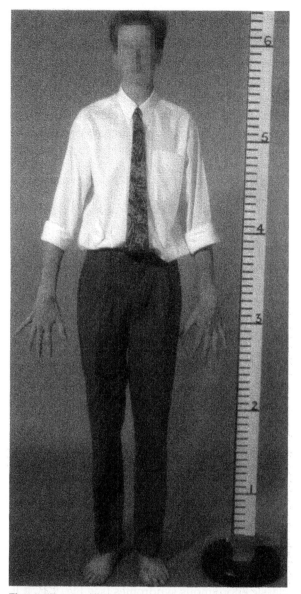

Figure 2.2 A patient showing the features of the marfanoid habitus. Note the height and the disproportionately long extremities

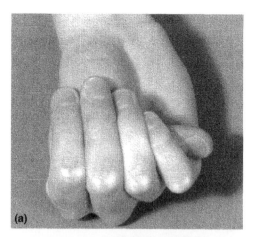

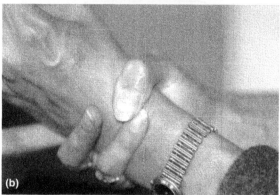

Figure 2.3 (a) The Steinberg test for arachnodactyly. It is possible to adduct the thumb across the palm so that it projects beyond the ulnar border of the hand. (b) The wrist sign for arachnodactyly. It is possible for the thumb and little finger (pinky) to meet around the wrist and overlap to the extent of a fingernail length. The test depends on the length of the digits, coupled with the slenderness of the wrist

---

Box 2.3 The characteristic features of the marfanoid habitus and the measurements on which its recognition is based

- Arachnodactyly (+ve Steinberg and wrist signs)
- High-arched palate
- Scoliosis, pectus deformity
- Span:height ratio > 1.03
- Upper segment:lower segment ratio < 0.89
- Hand:height ratio > 11%
- Foot:height ratio > 15%

---

decades ago the life expectancy of a person with MFS was 40 years. A combination of the use of serial echocardiography to monitor the aortic root diameter, the avoidance of contact sports and activities involving aerobic effort, β-blockers to lower blood pressure and improvements in aortic graft surgery has increased this to 70 years. In one recent study the 10-year survival rate was 75% in adults and 78% in children (Gillinov et al. 1997, Mingke et al. 1998). Close supervision during pregnancy is particularly important and frequent echocardiography is advised.

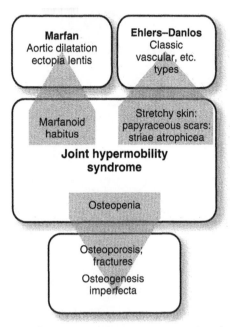

Figure 2.4 The relationship between JHS and its sister HDCTs and the overlap features that they share. Because both MFS and JHS share the marfanoid habitus their distinction relies on the presence or absence of aortic root dilatation and ectopia lentis, whose presence is identified by echocardiography and ophthalmic slit-lamp examination, respectively, hence the pivotal role played by these two investigations in the differential diagnosis

In spite of improvements in medicine and surgery, many patients with MFS die needlessly and prematurely because their condition has not been identified; their true diagnosis has gone by default and appropriate therapeutic action not been taken. Because the physiotherapist may be the first health professional to come into professional contact with such a patient, it behoves him or her to be alert to the possibility of undiagnosed MFS.

At the same time, it is important to appreciate that marfanoid habitus is not pathognomonic for MFS, as it is seen as part of many phenotypically related HDCTs, including JHS patients, among whom it is present in about one-third of cases (Grahame et al. 1981). The pivotal role of echocardiography and slit-lamp examination of the eye in clarifying the diagnosis of MFS is illustrated in Figure 2.4.

Ehlers–Danlos syndrome (EDS)

EDS is not a single disease but rather a group of some 10 related disorders, the common theme being a combination of joint hypermobility and hyperextensible (stretchy) skin. The current classification is the 'Villefranche Criteria' (Beighton et al. 1998a) (Table 2.5), which succeeded in simplifying the earlier Berlin Nosology (Beighton and De Paepe 1988).

Ehlers–Danlos syndrome – classic type

The classic form (formerly EDS types I and II) (see Table 2.2) is characterized by more spectacular degrees of hypermobility (Fig. 2.5) and subluxation (Fig. 2.6), and deformities are more pronounced (Fig. 2.7). Likewise, skin stretchiness is more obvious than that seen in the hypermobility type (EDS III, JHS) (Fig. 2.8) and the skin scars are more wrinkled, wide and gaping, and often violaceous in colour (Fig. 2.9) than those seen in JHS (Figs 2.10 and 2.11). The evidence is that classic EDS is caused by mutations in collagen type 5 (*COL51A*) (Burrows et al. 1997, De Paepe et al. 1997).

Ehlers–Danlos syndrome – hypermobility type

The hypermobility form of Ehlers–Danlos syndrome (formerly EDS type III) will be considered below under JHS. JHS is seen as a *forme fruste* of an HDCT, sharing clinical overlap with MFS, EDS and OI, but usually in a milder form than in the classic eponymous syndromes (see Fig. 2.4). It is now believed by many authorities, as seen from the hospital clinic perspective, to be identical to EDS hypermobility type (formerly EDS III) (Grahame 1999). Skin features are visible if sought, and comprise increased skin hyperextensibility (Fig. 2.8), impaired scar formation (Fig. 2.9) and striae (stretch marks). Striae atrophicae are seen in JHS often at sites and at times where and when one would not expect to see them. They are often most prominent over the thighs in non-obese adolescent girls, and in

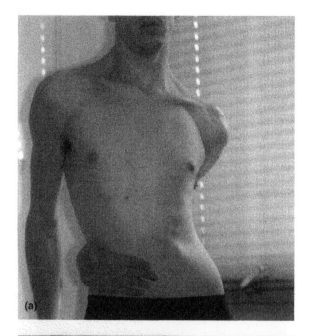

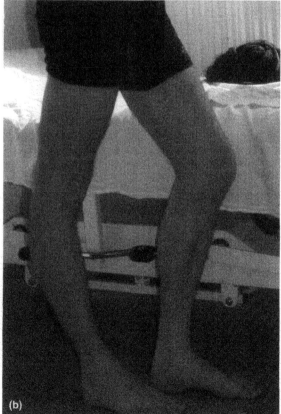

Figure 2.5 In EDS classic type the degree of joint laxity is greater than that seen in JHS/EDS hypermobility type

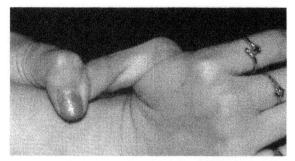

Figure 2.6 In EDS classic type the degree of joint instability and the resultant subluxation is greater than that seen in JHS/EDS hypermobility type

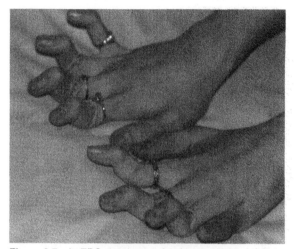

Figure 2.7 In EDS classic type the degree of joint deformity is greater than that seen in JHS/EDS hypermobility type

adults of all ages across the lumbar region (Fig. 2.12). Paradoxically, striae gravidarum are either exaggerated or absent altogether.

Ehlers–Danlos syndrome – vascular type

Unlike other types, the rarer vascular type (formerly EDS type IV) carries a poor prognosis as it may give rise to arterial, bowel or uterine rupture, with attendant dire consequences. These complications tend to occur between the ages of 20 and 40 years. It results from mutations in the gene for type III procollagen (*COL3A1*). In a recent study of 220 biochemically proven patients and 199 of their affected relatives, the median survival was 48 years (Pepin et al. 2000). Most deaths resulted from arterial rupture.

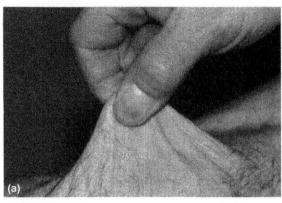

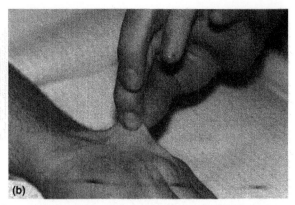

Figure 2.8   In EDS classic type the degree of skin stretch (hyperextensibility) (a) is greater than that seen in JHS/EDS hypermobility type (b)

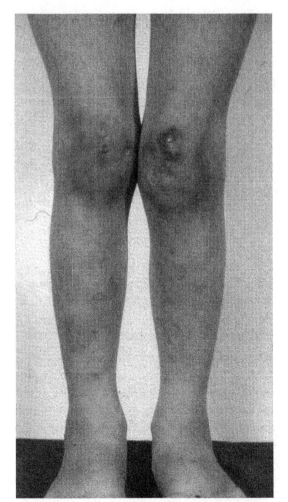

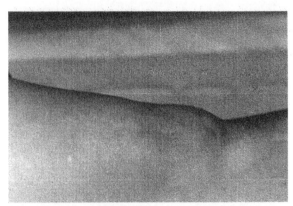

Figure 2.10   In JHS/EDS hypermobility type scar formation is also impaired but the scar tissue is visibly thin and fine. They provide good evidence that a connective tissue disorder is present and that the skin is involved

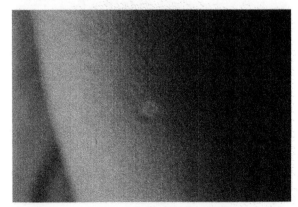

Figure 2.9   In EDS classic type scars tend to be of the wide and unsightly variety and papyraceous (paper-like). They often have a violaceous hue

Figure 2.11   A BCG inoculation scar is a good place to look for evidence of skin involvement in the JHS/EDS hypermobility type if the patient has had no surgical operations

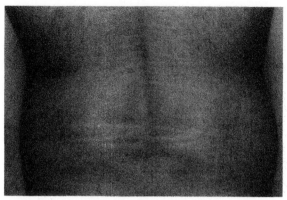

Figure 2.12 Striae atrophicae (stretch marks) provide another source of evidence that there is skin involvement in the JHS/EDS hypermobility type. They tend to appear in adolescent girls within a couple of years of the menarche, over the thighs and lumbar region

Ehlers–Danlos syndrome – other types

For more details the reader is referred to OMIM – Online Mendelian Inheritance in Man – see references.

To complete the description of EDS mention should be made of:

- Kyphoscoliosis and eye involvement type (EDS type VI)
- Arthrochalasis multiplex congenita (VIIa, dominant)
- Dermatosparaxis type (EDS type VII b,c, recessive)
- Periodontitis type (EDS type VIII)
- Progeroid type
- EDS, X-linked form with MVP and arterial rupture (type V)
- Recessive fibronectin defect type with abnormal platelet aggregation (type X)
- EDS due to tenascin-X deficiency.

It should be emphasized that these are rare variants.

Osteogenesis imperfecta (OI)

This is a hereditary form of osteoporosis caused by a mutation in either of the collagen 1 genes (*COL1A1* and *COL1A2*). The effect is to produce

brittle bones (which tend to fracture repeatedly on minimal provocation) and blue sclerae. Hypermobility is a recognized feature of OI. The clinical features are summarized in Table 2.3. The current classification is that of Byers, modified by Sillence (Byers 1993).

Joint hypermobility syndrome

Joint hypermobility syndrome (JHS) is the commonest of all the HDCTs and the one that occurs most frequently in clinical practice. JHS shares overlap features with the other HDCTs, including joint hypermobility, hyperextensible skin, impaired scar formation and striae atrophicae, the marfanoid habitus and, sometimes, osteopenia (Fig. 2.4) (Table 2.4). This has led to the notion that JHS is itself an (albeit mild) form of HDCT and that it and the hypermobile form of EDS (formerly known as EDS type III) are one and the same (Grahame 2000a). Unlike some of the better-known (though rarer) HDCTs it does not reduce life expectancy, but it carries with it the greatest burden of pain and disability (Grahame 2000b). It is considered in depth in Chapter 1.

GUIDELINES FOR REFERRAL FOR SPECIALIST MEDICAL ADVICE

There are situations when a physiotherapist will want to advise the patient to seek expert medical advice when confronted with signs of an HDCT. These will include:

- Where there is a complex array of clinical problems, acute and chronic, that may extend beyond the boundaries of the musculoskeletal system, where a comprehensive assessment is needed before embarking on a clearly targeted holistic treatment plan;
- Where the diagnosis of benign hypermobility (JHS) is uncertain because:
  — there are overlap features such as the marfanoid habitus;

— the patient has cardiorespiratory symptoms such as dyspnoea, chest pain or palpitation;

— there is a family history of Marfan syndrome and/or sudden cardiac death at an early age;

- Where the patient's symptoms do not match the physical findings:
  — The pain is disproportionate (excessive) taking into consideration the lack of signs of inflammation (swelling, redness, tenderness, loss of range), deformity, dislocation or subluxation;
  — There are areas of local tenderness reminiscent of fibromyalgia;
  — Excessive tiredness or fatigue;
  — Overt depression, anxiety or other manifestations of psychological distress;
  — Systemic symptoms such as fainting or orthostatic hypotension, suggesting autonomic dysfunction.
- When further investigations may be needed. These include:
  — Echocardiography and/or slit-lamp (ophthalmic) examination where MFS or other HDCTs are suspected (see under Marfan syndrome above);
  — Radiological investigation of:
    - Peripheral joints
    - Spine plain X-ray, CT scan or MRI to delineate spinal pathology.

GENETIC TESTING

At present there is a limited availability of laboratory tests that are of practical use in delineating the HDCTs or in distinguishing one from another. These investigations are labour-intensive and expensive, and few laboratories in the UK are suitably equipped to perform them. Most work is undertaken under the auspices of research grants and diagnostic applications are considered a secondary issue at best. Genetic testing for the HDCTs is in its infancy. The exciting discovery barely 15 years ago that mutations in the fibrillin-1 (*FBN1*) gene were the cause of Marfan syndrome, and the early promise of a simple diagnostic test for the disease, gave place to bitter disappointment when it became clear that over 200 such mutations were discovered in Marfan syndrome – almost one for every family investigated. However, in families with known mutations it is possible to use this knowledge to test family members in order to ascertain whether a particular individual has the mutation. No doubt as the science of molecular biology advances, the prospects for a laboratory-based diagnosis for the HDCTs using genetic methods will improve. In the meantime diagnosis rests on the use of validated clinical criteria (Beighton et al. 1988a, De Paepe et al. 1996; Beighton and De Paepe 1996, Grahame et al. 2000).

REFERENCES

Beighton, P., De Paepe, A., Steinmann, B. et al. (1998) Ehlers–Danlos syndromes: revised nosology, Villefranche, 1997. *American Journal of Medical Genetics*, **77**, 31–7.

Beighton, P., De Paepe, A., Danks, G. et al. (1988) International nosology of heritable disorders of connective tissue, Berlin 1986. *American Journal of Human Genetics*, **29**, 581–94.

Burrows, N.P., Nicholls, A.C., Yates, J.R. et al. (1997) Genetic linkage to the collagen alpha 1 (V) gene (*COL5A1*) in two British Ehlers–Danlos syndrome families with variable type I and II phenotypes. *Clinical and Experimental Dermatology*, **22**, 174–6.

Byers, P.H. (1993) Osteogenesis imperfecta. In: *Connective Tissue and its Heritable Disorders*. (P.L.S.B. Royce, ed.), pp. 317–50, Wiley-Liss.

De Paepe, A., Devereux, R.B., Dietz, H.C. et al. (1996) Revised diagnostic criteria for the Marfan syndrome. *American Journal of Medical Genetics*, **62**, 417–26.

De Paepe, A., Nuytinck, L., Hausser, I. et al. (1997) Mutations in the *COL5A1* gene are causal in the

Ehlers–Danlos syndromes I and II. *American Journal of Human Genetics*, **60**, 547–54.

Gillinov, A.M., Zehr, K.J., Redmond, J.M. et al. (1997) Cardiac operations in children with Marfan's syndrome: indications and results. *Annals of Thoracic Surgery*, **64**, 1140–4.

Grahame, R. (1999) Joint hypermobility and genetic collagen disorders: are they related? *Archives of Disease in Childhood*, **80**, 188–91.

Grahame, R. (2000a) Heritable disorders of connective tissue. In: *Baillière's Best Practice and Research in Clinical Rheumatology. Uncommon Non-inflammatory Osteoarticular Disorders.* Vol 14, No. 2. (Balint, G. and Bardin, T., eds), pp. 345–61, Baillière Tindall.

Grahame, R. (2000b) Pain, distress and joint hyperlaxity. *Joint Bone Spine*, **67**, 157–63.

Grahame, R., Edwards, J.C., Pitcher, D. et al. (1981) A clinical and echocardiographic study of patients with the hypermobility syndrome. *Annals of the Rheumatic Diseases*, **40**, 541–6.

Grahame, R., Bird, H.A., Child, A. et al. (2000) The British Society Special Interest Group on Heritable Disorders of Connective Tissue Criteria for the Benign Joint Hypermobility Syndrome. The Revised (Brighton 1998) Criteria for the Diagnosis of the BJHS. *Journal of Rheumatology*, **27**, 1777–9.

Mingke, D., Dresler, C., Pethig, K. et al. (1998) Surgical treatment of Marfan patients with aneurysms and dissection of the proximal aorta. *Journal of Cardiovascular Surgery*, **39**, 65–74.

OMIM classification (Online Mendelian Inheritance in Man). National Center for Biotechnology Information, USA (website http://www.ncbi.nlm. nih.gov/ Omim/searchomim.html)

Pepin, M., Schwarze, U., Superit-Furga, A. and Byers, P. (2000) Clinical and genetic features of Ehlers–Danlos syndrome type IV, the vascular type. *New England Journal of Medicine*, **342**, 673–80.

3

Overall management of the joint hypermobility syndrome

Rodney Grahame

Aims
This chapter aims to portray the overall management into which the subsequent chapters devoted to various aspects of physiotherapy management can be integrated. It is important for the therapist to be aware of the potential contribution to the management of JHS that can be offered by other members of the healthcare team, including rheumatologists, orthopaedic surgeons as well as occupational therapy, podiatry and pain management and self-help groups. The importance of assembling a management plan based on a multidisciplinary assessment is emphasized in order for the patient to benefit from all the potential help available.

This chapter sets out to take a bird's-eye view of the various modalities of treatment available for patients suffering from JHS. The approach is necessarily a multidisciplinary one but is unashamedly holistic in its philosophy. It is based on the approach used in the hypermobility clinics established by the author at the University College London Hospitals and the Great Ormond Children's Hospital in London since 1998.

Because of the ubiquitous nature of connective tissue proteins, the possible consequences of tissue trauma are legion. No two patients with JHS will present in an identical fashion. It follows that every patient will need a treatment plan tailored to his or her particular set of problems.

TREAT THE TREATABLE PRESENTING LESION(S)

Many of the musculoskeletal or articular lesions with which patients present are easily identifiable common conditions to which we all may fall prey (Beighton et al. 1999). Hypermobile subjects differ from other people in that their connective tissue defect renders them particularly vulnerable to the effects of trauma and overuse. Hence soft tissue injuries and stress fractures occur with greater frequency than in other people. The aim is to identify and assess all musculoskeletal lesions, past and present.

Soft tissue injury

The treatment of soft tissue lesions is generally along conventional lines with rest, physiotherapy, local steroid injections and surgery as appropriate. There are, however, a number of caveats that relate to the specific situation that may modify their use.

Rest

In the treatment of acute injury rest should be prescribed prudently in one whose musculature may have become deconditioned as a result of fear of the pain that movement will induce. The handling of trauma-vulnerable tissues is of particular importance to physiotherapists and other manual therapists confronted by patients presenting with soft tissue lesions (see Chapter 7). The use of therapeutic techniques that promote healing, such as massage and ultrasound, is indicated but should be moderate.

Local steroid injections

One of the inevitable consequences of a tissue laxity syndrome where collagen is deficient or defective is that healing is delayed and often incomplete. This applies to the formation of scars following surgery or injury, but it also applies to spontaneous recovery from chronic injury or overuse lesions, such as muscle and ligament tears,

tenosynovitis, and lesions of the enthesis (sites of tendon–bone insertion), such as epicondylitis or plantar fasciitis. From Chapter 1 it will be clear that many of the common presentations of JHS fall within this category. In most, the accepted approach is to administer a local corticosteroid infiltration (hydrocortisone acetate mixed with lignocaine 1% is a widely used preparation). However, corticosteroids are potent inhibitors of collagen synthesis by fibroblasts, and thus their use is accompanied by the possibility of aggravating a fraught situation further. This does not mean that local steroid injections are totally contraindicated (although it is prudent always to consider the use of physical treatments first). Because the protein synthesis-inhibiting effect is dose related (Harvey and Grahame 1973) one strategy is to use the minimal possible effective dose while taking the necessary precaution of targeting the injection as accurately as possible to the precise site of the lesion. Another is to avoid the use of depo steroid preparations (such as methylprednisolone (Depo-Medrone) or triamcinolone hexacetonide (Lederspan) or acetonide (Kenalog), and to ensure the exclusive use of soluble preparations such as hydrocortisone acetate (Hydrocortistab).

Surgery

Surgery is another therapeutic modality, which should not be undertaken lightly and then only after weighing the benefits against the risk of failure (see case history at end of chapter). The results of surgical operations in JHS patients are often disappointing both to the patient and the surgeon (Finsterbush and Pogrund 1982). This is particularly evident in relation to orthopaedic procedures, such as operations to relieve chondromalacia patellae and recurrent dislocation of the patella or shoulder, which are frequently undertaken on JHS patients. The basic problem is threefold: first, that tissues are less robust than normal and are less amenable to surgical procedures, and there is a tendency to unsightly scar formation (Fig. 3.1) and for sutures to tear through, leading to dehiscence of the wound (Fig. 3.2). Secondly,

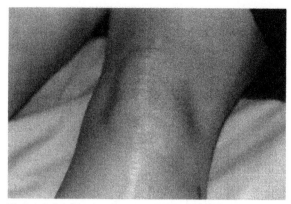

Figure 3.1   An unsightly operative scar following an operation to realign the patellar ligament in a patient with JHS

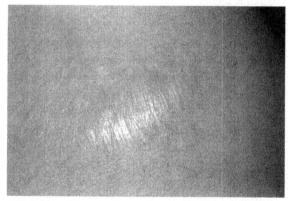

Figure 3.2   A surgical wound that has dehisced, leaving a large area of fine and thin scar tissue in a patient with JHS

the fragility and friability of blood vessels can cause technical problems with wound closure and haemostasis during operations (Beighton and Horan 1969). Thirdly, as stated above, healing tends to be delayed and may be incomplete. None of these considerations necessarily renders JHS a contraindication to surgery. Provided the surgeon is aware that the patient has a tissue laxity diathesis, and provided that he or she is prepared to recognize and acknowledge it, a mere adaptation of technique is all that is required.

A different situation arises in the case of Ehlers–Danlos syndrome vascular type (EDS IV), where the blood vessels, viscera and other tissues are excessively fragile and any surgical or interventional radiological procedure carries a high risk of tissue or vascular damage and wound dehiscence (Berney et al. 1994).

Physiotherapy

Physiotherapy in its various modalities (general advice, passive mobilization, exercise therapy, joint stabilization procedures, proprioceptive enhancement, rehabilitation and chronic pain management) forms the mainstay of treatment and will be covered in depth in later chapters.

Podiatry

The majority of JHS patients, both adults and children, have flat feet, although many are not aware of it. The characteristic feature is that while the foot is non-weight bearing it presents a normal appearance with a full (sometimes exaggerated) longitudinal arch, which flattens out immediately it bears the body's weight. At the same time the foot tends to become pronated. The result is the classic JHS flat foot (see Fig. 1.2d). Milder forms cause little in the way of symptoms and can be ignored, whereas more severe cases should be assessed by a podiatrist, who can measure the patient and recommend suitable orthoses.

Computerized gait analysis providing pressure and force/time information is now available and is capable of providing precise understanding of the biomechanics of gait in hypermobile individuals (Fig. 3.3).

Occupational therapy

The potential role of occupational therapy in the treatment of JHS is considerable, but it is one that has as yet to be fully explored. As will be clear from a perusal of several of the following chapters, people with JHS often have great practical problems in performing their tasks at work, in school or college, in the home, or when at leisure. Occupational therapists can contribute in a major way to making people's immediate living and working environment more user friendly. Their input into this area of rehabilitation is long overdue.

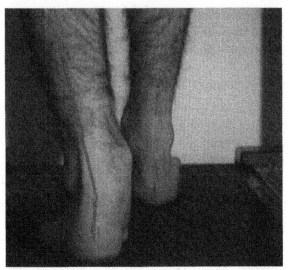

Figure 3.3 Computerized gait analysis (podiatric kinematic visualization) showing abnormal propulsive pronation with marked Helbig's sign (bowing of the tendo Achilles) in a 29-year-old male patient with JHS. With thanks to Mr Ron McCulloch of the London Podiatric Centre

Prolotherapy

The definition of prolotherapy (formerly known as sclerotherapy) is the injection of a material in solution with the aim of tightening and strengthening loose or weak tendons, ligaments or joint capsules through the activation of fibroblasts to produce collagen (Reeves 1995). The most widely used agents are 15% dextrose solution and sodium morrhuate. Widely promoted in the USA for the treatment of low back pain, there have been anecdotal claims by individual JHS patients of benefit from this form of therapy. Thus far there are no published reports of scientific evidence for its efficacy in JHS.

MANAGING PAIN

Mild pain

Analgesic drugs are widely used by JHS patients. Mild pain can be helped by paracetamol or non-steroidal anti-inflammatory drugs (NSAIDs).

The conventional NSAIDs, known as Cox 1 drugs, which include aspirin, naproxen and diclofenac, have the potential to cause gastric side-effects. Recently introduced, the equipotent Cox 2 NSAIDs such as celecoxib, rofecoxib, nabumetone and etoricoxib are reported to have a less irritant effect on the stomach.

Moderate pain

Moderately severe pain may require one of the weak opioid drugs such as co-proxamol, dihydrocodeine or codeine phosphate.

Severe pain

The use of potent opioids such as morphine, oxycodone, fentanyl, buprenorphine, dextromoramide, hydromorphone and methadone in musculoskeletal disorders is inadvisable except in exceptional circumstances during an acute painful crisis, and only when other agents have been tried and found wanting.

Chronic pain

Caution is advised in relying on the analgesics and NSAIDs, which, though helpful in the short term in tiding the patient over acute painful episodes, are disappointingly ineffective in chronic pain. Furthermore, they carry the risk of potentially serious side-effects, in particular gastrointestinal bleeding. JHS patients with chronic pain report that their pain is resistant to maximum doses of even potent analgesic drugs such as those listed above. This tendency should be resisted, as habituation will rapidly follow with little to show for it in terms of pain relief. The basis for this resistance to pain control in the face of conventional potent analgesics is not known, but suggests a possible defect in pain processing, one of a number of neurophysiological abnormalities recently discovered to be present in patients with JHS (see Chapter 1). By contrast, alternative pain-relieving options, such as the use of low-dose (5–10 mg at bedtime) amitriptyline (a tricyclic antidepressant) or the application of transcutaneous electrical nerve stimulation (TENS), can be very helpful where other methods fail.

Local anaesthetics

JHS patients should be warned that local anaesthetic injections are less effective than in other people, and this can cause distress to patients and consternation among clinicians when such means of analgesia are used, e.g. in the course of dental or other minor surgery, or with the use of epidural anaesthesia during childbirth (see Chapter 1) (Arendt-Nielsen et al. 1990).

Pain management programmes

When a chronic pain syndrome becomes established and the quality of life starts to diminish, then little short of a full pain management programme using cognitive behavioural techniques can restore JHS patients to anything like their former function. The use of these techniques is discussed in detail in Chapter 10.

SELF-HELP

As stated in Chapter 1, every person with JHS has his or her own unique variation of the condition and no-one understands its nuances better than the individuals themselves. It follows that no-one is better placed to manage the condition throughout its various crises and vicissitudes. But competence in self-management does not come naturally: it derives from knowledge of the disease, its treatment, and of one's own personal characteristics. This applies to any number of the various acute lesions referred to above.

In the absence of any such identifiable lesions the precise reason for the distressing and widespread diffuse musculoskeletal pain may elude

patients with hypermobility. However, many can often identify exacerbating and relieving factors. Unaccustomed physical exercise is the usual trigger, and patients can usually recognize the limits beyond which they can expect to suffer increased levels of pain. This may relate to a change in job, a leisure activity or a rapid weight gain. In many cases lifestyle modification in the right direction can both prevent and relieve pain.

Self-help groups set up by people with HDCTs for patients with HDCTs play an important role in providing information and support for their members by providing leaflets, books and newsletters, holding study days and maintaining interactive web sites. In the UK there are active groups catering for people with HDCTs. Details of the Hypermobility Syndrome Association are provided in Chapter 11.

For further reading on the general aspects of the management in JHS the reader is referred to Beighton et al. 1999 and Grahame 2000.

Illustrative case history

A 34-year-old teacher, an enthusiastic gymnast, a talented musician (piano and clarinet) and singer, presented with the following history. At the age of 18 she developed painful unstable knees. For some reason she followed a surgical route and proceeded to undergo no fewer than 10 operations on her knees over the subsequent 17 years (five on the right, five on the left). Each successive operation was performed by a different surgeon, who attempted to improve on the indifferent result achieved by his predecessor. At the end of this time the patient was noted to be hypermobile, but the full significance of this observation was unappreciated. An eleventh operation was performed 5 years later. Two years after this a definitive diagnosis of JHS/EDS III was confirmed by a clinical geneticist. She remains severely disabled, using elbow crutches because of an unstable right knee, and is dependent on opiates for pain relief. She was forced to seek medical retirement from her teaching job and is no longer able to participate in her physical or musical activities.

The moral of this cautionary tale is that patients with JHS do not generally respond well to surgical interventions, and conservative methods should always be adopted in preference to surgery in the first instance, along the lines detailed in the various chapters of this book. An exclusively surgical approach is not to be recommended for JHS patients.

REFERENCES

Arendt-Nielsen, L., Kaalund, P., Bjerring, P. and Hogsaa, B. (1990) Insufficient effect of local analgesics in Ehlers–Danlos type III patients (connective tissue disorder). *Acta Anaesthesiologica Scandinavica*, **34**, 358–61.

Beighton, P.H., Grahame, R. and Bird, H.A. (1999) *Hypermobility of Joints*, 3rd edn. Springer-Verlag.

Beighton, P. and Horan, F. (1969) Orthopaedic aspects of the Ehlers–Danlos syndrome. *Journal of Bone and Joint Surgery*, **51B**, 446–52.

Berney, T., La Scala, G. and Vettoral, D. et al. (1994) Surgical pitfalls in a patient with type IV Ehlers–Danlos syndrome and colonic rupture. *Surgery Colon Rectum*, **37**, 1038–42.

Finsterbush, A. and Pogrund, H. (1982) The hypermobility syndrome. Musculoskeletal complaints in 100 consecutive cases of generalised joint hypermobility. *Clinical Orthopedics*, **168**, 124–7.

Grahame, R. (2000) Heritable disorders of connective tissue. *Best Practice and Research in Clinical Rheumatology*, **14**, 345–61.

Harvey, W. and Grahame, R. (1973) Effect of some adrenal steroid hormones on skin fibroblast replication in vitro. *Annals of the Rheumatic Diseases*, **32**, 272.

Reeves, K.D. (1995) Prolotherapy. Present and future applications in soft-tissue pain and disability. *Physical Medicine and Rehabilitation Clinics of North America*, **6**, 917.

4

Hypermobility syndrome in children

Susan Maillard
Kevin J. Murray

Aims

1. To describe the different clinical conditions and phenomena that occur in children with joint hypermobility
2. To describe how JHS presents in children
3. To discuss the multidisciplinary management of JHS

Joint hypermobility is understood to result from either genetic defects or variations in connective tissue matrix proteins, which results in more extensible tissues. Some authors describe this heterogeneous group as the heritable disorders of connective tissue (HDCT) (Grahame 1999). Within this group are disorders such as Ehlers–Danlos syndrome, Marfan syndrome and osteogenesis imperfecta. All these genetic connective tissue disorders have hypermobility as a feature, but hypermobility is also relatively common within the general population and may be a result of more common genetic variations rather than mutations as such (Grahame 2000).

PATHOPHYSIOLOGY

Joint hypermobility syndrome appears to be inherited as a gender-influenced dominant trait (Beighton et al. 1988, Beighton and Horan 1970, Carter and Wilkinson 1964, Child 1986, Grahame 2000, Henney et al. 1992, Horton et al. 1980, Jessee et al. 1980). It has not been possible to identify a single gene abnormality, but some variation in collagen type I/type III ratios have been observed. However, it may be more likely that the condition represents a complex genetic trait whereby multiple genes influence the phenotype of the individual.

Type I collagen is the most common collagen in the human body and is abundant in connective tissues such as tendon, ligament, joint capsule, skin, demineralized bone and nerve receptors. Type III is also present to a lesser extent in these structures, and type II is found predominantly in hyaline cartilage. Type III is thin and elastic and found in relatively greater amounts in extensible connective tissue, such as the lungs, skin and vascular system (Child 1986, Handler et al. 1985, Prockop and Kivirikko 1995). In children with hypermobility the ratio of type III collagen to type III + type I is increased (El-Shahaly and El-Sherif 1991), and this is thought to underlie the increased tissue flexibility of childhood (or loss of it with ageing).

Neurological structures or tissues may also be affected, which is indicated by the increased incidence of acroparaesthesia (abnormal sensations in hands and feet) in children with JHS. There is also evidence that proprioception and joint spatial awareness are reduced, particularly at the end of the range of movement of the joints (Hall et al. 1995, Mallik et al. 1994). Further research indicates a poor response to local anaesthesia in some individuals, and there is also a connection between benign congenital hypotonia and ligamentous laxity in the floppy infant.

PAEDIATRIC CONDITIONS WITH HYPERMOBILITY AS A CLINICAL FINDING

As in many aspects of paediatric medicine, all possible causes must have been considered before a diagnosis of JHS can be made (Box 4.1). The degree of hypermobility will vary from global to localized. Specific genetic disorders that

---

Box 4.1 Definable clinical conditions which have been associated with joint hypermobility as a clinical finding

Achondroplasia (Raff and Byers 1996)
Clumsy children
Congenital hip dysplasia (Gulan et al. 2000, Hamilton and Broughton 1998, Wenger and Frick 1999)
Congenital hip dislocation (Carter and Wilkinson 1964)
Chondromalacia patellae (Al-Rawi and Nessan 1997, Lewkonia and Ansell 1983)
Down syndrome
Dyspraxia
Ehlers–Danlos syndrome (Dolan et al. 1998)
Fibromyalgia (Bridges et al. 1992, El-Shahaly and El Sherif 1991, Gedalia et al. 1993b, Goldman 1991, Hudson et al. 1995)
Growing pains = benign paroxymal nocturnal leg pains
Infantile hypotonia
Juvenile episodic arthralgias of childhood
Larsen syndrome (Raff and Byers 1996)
Marfan syndrome (Lannoo et al. 1996)
Morquio syndrome (Raff and Byers 1996)
Motor developmental delay (Davidovitch et al. 1994, Jaffe et al. 1988, Russek 1999, Tirosh et al. 1991)
Osteogenesis imperfecta (Engelbert et al. 1999)
Spondylolysis/spondylolythesis
Stickler syndrome
Trichorhinopharyngeal syndrome

---

cause hypermobility in childhood include:

1. **Ehlers–Danlos syndrome.** All forms of this syndrome cause clinical problems, such as skin fragility, unsightly bruising and scarring, musculoskeletal discomfort due to recurrent sprains, subluxations and dislocations, and an increased susceptibility to osteoarthritis. One form that is potentially fatal is termed Ehlers–Danlos vascular type (formerly EDS type IV), which predominantly involves vascular structures, and death results from the rupture of arteries, bowel or other large organs (Pepin et al. 2000, Pyeritz 2000).

2. **Osteogenesis imperfecta (OI).** There are several forms of this condition, all of which have a varying degree of hypermobility associated with them. However, research indicates that among children with OI, those with generalized joint hypermobility are less likely to develop scoliosis and occipitobasilar impression (Engelbert et al. 1998).

3. **Stickler syndrome**. Stickler syndrome is an autosomal dominant disorder with characteristic ophthalmological and orofacial features, deafness and arthritis. These children typically have a flat midface with a depressed nasal bridge, short nose, anteverted nares, micrognathia and severe myopia. Retinal detachment may lead to blindness. There is generalized joint hypermobility, which often disappears with age, and mild to severe osteoarthritis that typically develops in the third or fourth decade. Mild spondyloepiphyseal dysplasia (specific progressive changes in bone and joint formation due to a genetic mutation) is often apparent radiologically (Snead and Yates 1999).

4. **Marfan syndrome**. Marfan syndrome is an autosomal dominant genetic disorder caused by a defect in the gene which encodes for a specific protein, Fibrillin 1 (*FBN1*). Such individuals present with a characteristically tall stature, long limbs (where the arm span:height ratio exceeds 1.03), little subcutaneous fat and muscle hypotonia. There may also be complications with the cardiovascular system and the eyes (see Chapter 2). Joint hypermobility can be recognized in as many as 85% of children with Marfan syndrome (Grahame and Pyeritz 1995, Lannoo et al. 1996).

There are other recognized clinical features that are closely associated with hypermobility. These include:

1. **Anterior knee pain**. Generalized joint laxity, and particularly hypermobility of the knee, is considered a possible contributing factor in the development of anterior knee pain and chondromalacia patellae (Al-Rawi and Nessan 1997). These authors also found that chondromalacia patellae was associated with wasting of the quadriceps muscle and with flat feet and backache, the latter two also commonly associated with generalized joint hypermobility.

2. **Motor development delay**. Hypermobility can be evident as early as infancy. There is said to be a higher incidence of both gross and fine motor delay in children who are hypermobile, even in the absence of an identified neurological deficit (Jaffe et al. 1988, Tirosh et al. 1991) (see p 38).

3. **Fibromyalgia**. See under chronic pain syndromes (p 39).

JOINT HYPERMOBILITY SYNDROME IN CHILDREN

Joint hypermobility syndrome is diagnosed when hypermobility becomes symptomatic and when other heritable disorders of connective tissue and other causes of the symptoms have been considered and ruled out.

Diagnosis and assessment

There have been many scoring systems devised for measuring or defining hypermobility. The first, proposed by Carter and Wilkinson (1964) was then modified by Beighton et al. (1973). The Beighton scoring system has proved the most popular worldwide. There is also a scale devised by Rotés that is used in most Spanish-speaking countries, which adds more items of clinical interest (quoted in Bulbena et al. 1992). Table 4.1 lists the three different scoring criteria. The different systems differ slightly in their particular ways of assessing a joint. Together with these clinical manoeuvres, other instrumental methods to assess joint hypermobility have been used (Bulbena et al. 1992) i.e. clinical goniometers (Beighton et al. 1988, Mishra et al. 1996), fixed torque devices (Beighton et al. 1973) and hyper-extensometer (Bird et al. 1979). There is no universally accepted Beighton score required in order to accept a diagnosis of JHS in the presence of associated musculoskeletal symptoms. Some have taken 5/9, others 6/9.

Table 4.1 Comparisons of the different methods of measuring the hypermobility criteria: Carter and Wilkinson, Beighton and Rotés criteria (Bulbena et al. 1992)

Criteria	Carter and Wilkinson	Beighton et al.	Rotés
Thumb abduction	1	1*	1
Elbow extension >10°	1	1*	1
Finger extension >90° (metacarpophalangeal)	1	1*	1
Knee extension >10°	1	1*	1
Excess ROM ankle dorsiflexion and eversion	1		
Palms flat on floor		1	1
External shoulder rotation			1
Cervical rotation			1
Cervical side flexion			1
Hip abduction			1
Metatarsophalangeal >90°			1
Lumbar lateral hypermobility			1
Total score	**5**	**9**	**11**

*1 point each side.

Bulbena et al. (1992) compared the scales proposed by Carter and Wilkinson (1964), Beighton et al. (1973) and Rotés (quoted in Bulbena et al. 1992) and found a high correlation between the different scores, suggesting high concurrent and predictive validity. From this they proposed a set of criteria which they considered the best definition of hypermobility.

One intrinsic difficulty in measuring ranges of passive movement is that the observed range depends upon the force applied to the moving part, which may vary with the enthusiasm of the examiner and the pain threshold and cooperation of the child (Silverman et al. 1975). In children it is good practice to assess all joints for hypermobility initially in order to establish the degree of hypermobility, i.e. global or localized, as this will guide the treatment programme.

A set of classification criteria for **joint hypermobility syndrome** (as opposed to **hypermobility**), validated so far for adults only, was developed in Brighton in 1998 (Grahame et al. 2000).

Careful clinical evaluation and, where appropriate, laboratory tests, may be done to rule out other more serious conditions which may have similar symptoms, e.g. juvenile idiopathic arthritis (JIA) and other inflammatory polyarthritis conditions (Kirk et al. 1967), Ehlers–Danlos and Marfan syndrome. Findings of marked hyperelastic skin and lenticular abnormalities are not usually seen in JHS, but mild or moderate increases in skin stretchiness, hernias, relatively easy bruising and poor wound healing may be seen (El-Shahaly and El-Sherif 1991, Mishra et al. 1996), indicating some overlap with these well-defined genetic conditions.

In the assessment of a child with hypermobility it is important to assess the strength of muscles surrounding the joints, as well as the endurance of the muscles and the general stamina of the child. These factors are often reduced in JHS, and improving them will be an important part of the treatment programme. It is also important that balance and proprioception are assessed to determine their impact on the child's symptoms, and the management programme should address any deficiencies (Augustsson and Thomee 2000, Finsterbush and Pogrund 1982, Visser et al. 2000).

Prevalence of joint hypermobility

The reports of the prevalence of hypermobility must be viewed cautiously because of the variability in the diagnostic criteria used. Joint hypermobility has been reported in 6.7–43% of children (Table 4.2), depending upon age, ethnicity, and the criteria used to assess hypermobility. The prevalence is higher in girls: 7.1–57%, compared to 6.0–35% in boys (Decoster et al. 1997, Gedalia et al. 1985, Kerr et al. 2000, Russek 1999, Vougiouka et al. 2000). Given the high proportion of subjects documented as 'hypermobile' in some studies, it is clear that the different systems of assessment have major limitations in defining a cohort of hypermobile subjects at significant risk of musculoskeletal problems in different populations.

Table 4.2 Prevalence of joint hypermobility in different populations of children

Population	Reference	Criteria used	Age	No. of subjects	Total % hypermobile	No. of subjects F/M	% Male hypermobile	% Female hypermobile
British school children	Carter and Wilkinson, 1964	Carter–Wilkinson 4/5	6–11	285	6.7	140/145	6.2	7.1
US school children	Gedalia et al. 1985	Modified Beighton*	5–17	260	12.3	126/134	6.7	18.3
US adolescent athletes	Decoster et al. 1997	Beighton 5/9	15.5 avg.	264	12.9	114/150	6.0	21.9
US music students	Larsson et al. 1987	Beighton 3/9	14–68	660	19.1	300/360	6.9	33.7
Non-Caucasian Brazilian school children	Forleo et al. 1993	Carter–Wilkinson 5/9	5–17	416	31.7			
Brazilian school children	Forleo et al. 1993	Carter–Wilkinson 5/9	5–17	1005	36.3	560/445	33.7	38.4
Caucasian Brazilian school children	Forleo et al. 1993	Carter–Wilkinson 5/9	5–17	589	39.6			
Greek school children	Vougiouka et al. 2000	Beighton** 3/5	5–14	2432	8.8	1152/1280	7.1	10.8
Icelandic school children	Qvindesland et al. 1999	Beighton 4/9	12		26.7		12.9	40.5
People in Singapore	Seow et al. 1999	Modified Beighton*	15–39	306	17			
Dutch school children	Rikken-Bultman et al.1997	Beighton 5/9	4–13	252	15.5			
Dutch school children	Rikken-Bultman et al.1997	Beighton 5/9	12–17	658	13.4			
West African people	Birrell et al.1994	Beighton 4/9	6–66	204	43		35.0	57.0

* Criteria as in Beighton et al. except for hyperextension of fingers to lie parallel to forearm (as in Carter and Wilkinson) rather than hyperextension of fifth MCP joint to 90°.
** Scoring using the right limbs only and lumbar flexion.

Table 4.3 Prevalence of joint hypermobility in populations reporting chronic or recurrent joint or muscle pain, with no specific other rheumatic or musculoskeletal condition

Population	Criteria used	Reference	Age	Total no. with symptoms	Total % with symptoms
Israeli school children with JRA	Modified Beighton 3/5*	Gedalia et al. 1993	5–17	34	2.9
Paediatric rheumatology referrals	Beighton 3/5**	Biro et al. 1983	NK	262#	5.7
USA school children with episodic arthritis/arthralgia‡	Modified Beighton* 3/5	Gedalia et al. 1985,1988, Gedalia and Press 1998	5–17	32	65.6
Israeli children with fibromyalgia	Modified Beighton* 3/5	Gedalia et al. 1993	9–15	21	81.0
Arthralgia in US school children	NK	Arroyo et al. 1988	5–19	66	50
Greek school children	Beighton 3/5**	Vougiouka et al. 2000	5–14	189	21.2
Chondromalacia patellae and hypermobility	Beighton 4/9	Al-Rawi et al. 1997	10–29	115	81

* Criteria as in Beighton et al. except for hyperextension of fingers to lie parallel to forearm rather than hyperextension of the fifth MCP joint to 90°.
# 3/15 subjects were diagnosed with juvenile arthritis, leaving 12/262 or 4.6% with primary hypermobility syndrome.
‡ Specifically excluded children with juvenile idiopathic arthritis (JIA).
** Measured only the right limbs and lumbar flexion.

Hypermobility is also more prevalent among Asians than Africans, and more prevalent in Africans than Caucasians. However, it appears that hypermobility decreases with age (Acasuso-Diaz and Collantes-Estevez 1998, Birrell et al. 1994, Cheng et al. 1991, El-Garf et al. 1998, El-Shahaly and El-Sherif 1991, Hudson et al. 1998, Kirk et al. 1967, Russek 1999), and that far fewer adults are hypermobile compared to the number of hypermobile children.

Clinical presentation

Many children have hypermobile joints, but only a percentage of those will suffer from symptoms, and if they follow a chronic pattern these children are often diagnosed as having JHS (Grahame 1999). The symptoms and their severity will vary from child to child, and can occur at any age (Table 4.3). Children may present to an orthopaedic surgeon, rheumatologist, paediatric rheumatologist, paediatrician, general practitioner, physiotherapist or other manual therapist with any of a wide range of traumatic or non-traumatic painful complaints (Box 4.2).

These children typically lack the positive laboratory findings found in other rheumatological conditions and rarely develop any radiological abnormalities. Occasionally transient mild swelling or puffiness and, more rarely, joint effusions may occur, but normally only last for hours or very occasionally days (Kirk et al. 1967, Russek 1999, Scharf and Nahir 1982). The occurrence and location of symptoms are variable, but appear to be more common in the lower limbs.

In the very young child hypermobility may be detected with evidence of delayed motor development and a degree of clumsiness (Davidovitch, et al. 1994, Jaffe et al. 1988, Moreira and Wilson 1992, Tirosh et al. 1991). However, the motor delay is usually self-limiting if hypermobility is the only cause. This problem will either improve spontaneously or with a motor development rehabilitation programme. A number of parents of hypermobile children do report

---

Box 4.2 Neuromuscular and musculoskeletal complications or features seen in children with JHS

Acute or traumatic
Sprains (Grahame et al. 1981)
Strains – recurrent ankle strains (Finsterbush and Pogrund 1982)
    – knee, meniscus tears (Bulbena et al. 1992)
Acute or recurrent dislocations/subluxations, i.e.

- Shoulder joint (Finsterbush and Pogrund 1982)
- Patella (Biro et al. 1983, Finsterbush and Pogrund 1982, Runow 1983, Stanitski 1995)
- Metacarpophalangeal (MCP) joint

Traumatic arthritis/synovitis
Bruising (Bird et al. 1978, Bulbena et al. 1993)
Fractures (Grahame et al. 1981)

Chronic or non-traumatic
Soft-tissue rheumatism (El-Shahaly and El-Sherif 1991, Gedalia et al. 1985, Goldman 1991, Grahame et al. 1981, Hudson et al. 1995, Kirk et al. 1967)

- Tendonitis
- Synovitis
- Juvenile episodic arthritis/synovitis
- Bursitis

Anterior knee pain
Back pain – lumbar or thoracic (Al-Rawi and Nessan 1997, El-Shahaly and El-Sherif 1991, Grahame 1999, Howell 1984, Larsson et al. 1993, Larsson et al. 1995, Lewkonia and Ansell 1983)
Scoliosis (Bulbena et al. 1992, El-Shahaly and El-Sherif 1991, Finsterbush and Pogrund 1982)
Chronic widespread musculoskeletal pain syndromes
Nerve compression disorders (El-Shahaly and El-Sherif 1991)
Acroparaesthesia (Francis et al. 1987)

Flat feet and ankle/foot pain (Al-Rawi and Nessan 1997, Bulbena 1992, Finsterbush and Pogrund 1982)
Unspecified arthralgia or effusion of joints (Biro et al. 1983, El-Shahaly and El-Sherif 1991, Finsterbush and Pogrund 1982, Hudson et al. 1995, Kirk et al. 1967, Lewkonia and Ansell 1983)

---

ongoing clumsiness in their children well into later childhood.

There is no evidence to suggest that JHS is linked to more serious conditions of the cardiac system, bone, skin or eyes (Grahame et al. 2000, Mishra et al. 1996). However, the evidence linking hypermobility and pulled elbows is not clear, as some reports suggest there is a link whereas others have not found a correlation (Hagroo et al. 1995).

There is, however, evidence that links hypermobility to many other symptoms.

Lower limb arthralgia

Pain in the lower limbs may present as anterior knee pain, generalized knee pain and ankle/foot arthralgia. Children will often complain of pain after physical activity and towards the end of the day, and this may be due to muscular pain as well as joint pain. Early morning stiffness, stiffness after rest periods or prolonged stiffness, which are the hallmark of inflammatory rheumatic disorders, are less prominent in JHS-related problems (Arroyo et al. 1988, Bensahel et al. 2000, Grahame 2000, Hall et al. 1995, Kerr et al. 2000, Vougiouka et al. 2000).

It has been recognized that hypermobility may be a contributing factor in the pathogenesis of chondromalacia patellae, and that this may be associated with pain in the ankles, hips and back (Al-Rawi and Nessan 1997).

A number of children with a history of 'growing pains' or 'benign paroxysmal nocturnal leg pain' have been documented as having generalized hypermobility. Others who are diagnosed with a hypermobility problem or JHS in later life often recall a history of 'growing pains'. It is conceivable that these pains may be related to periods of unaccustomed excessive activity (such as after an intensive physical education (PE) lesson) in those predisposed by underlying hypermobility.

Back pain

Back pain in children and adolescents requires thorough investigation and assessment. However, one of the most common differential diagnoses is hypermobility (Grahame 1999, Scharf and Nahir 1982). This aspect affects adolescents most often, and may be related to a particular physical activity. Thus, hypermobility may affect the whole of the spine or a specific area only, and often results in an S-shaped posture with increased curves in the cervical, thoracic or lumbar regions. The pain is often associated with acute muscle spasm, and if not managed appropriately in the early stages may result in chronic back pain, continuing poor posture, and the associated difficulties that these bring. Poor sitting posture and the weight of the books carried at school often exacerbate this.

If the pain is severe, specific lesions seen more frequently in hypermobile children, need to be considered, such as spondylolysis, spondylolisthesis and, in older children, disc prolapse.

Chronic pain syndromes

There has been significant research establishing links between hypermobility and fibromyalgia. Fibromyalgia is a chronic pain syndrome associated with multiple muscle tenderness and localized tender points, marked sleep disturbance and high levels of disability. The results are inconclusive, but they do suggest an association between joint hypermobility and fibromyalgia in that there appears to be a high percentage of fibromyalgic children who are also hypermobile (Acasuso-Diaz and Collantes-Estevez 1998, Buskila et al. 1995, Gedalia et al. 1993, 2000).

A link has also been reported between hypermobility and the development of reflex sympathetic dystrophy (Francis et al. 1987, Murray and Woo 2001), and other localized chronic pain syndromes. Many children who present with these pain syndromes are also hypermobile, and it is very difficult to distinguish between the symptoms of JHS and chronic pain syndromes, which may complicate it.

In addition, it has been noted that adults with JHS are more likely to have anxiety disorders than a comparison group with other rheumatological conditions (Bulbena et al. 1993). It often becomes apparent that there is an element of pain amplification in children with JHS, and in these cases it is appropriate to consider a psychological approach to pain management as well as a physical approach.

Other symptoms

Although subluxations, dislocations, sprains, strains and other soft tissue rheumatic conditions are more common in children with JHS (Hudson et al. 1998) the resultant damage occurring with these acute injuries may, paradoxically, actually be decreased because of the increased laxity of joint structures, and the true recovery time thereby reduced. However, the increased frequency of occurrence in hypermobile children may add to the overall burden.

Many researchers have found a correlation between temporomandibular dysfunction (TMD) and hypermobility (Buckingham et al. 1991, Khan and Pedlar 1996, Perrini et al. 1997), though not uniformly (Conti et al. 2000, Khan and Pedlar 1996, Winocur et al. 2000). Symptoms of pain, subluxation and clicking in the temporomandibular joint have been reported.

Many of the childhood problems discussed above may persist well into adult life and require similar treatment methods.

Balance and proprioception

Children with hypermobility are reported by their parents to be clumsy or have generally poor balance. This is thought to be due in part to reduced proprioception in joints, most marked at the extremes of the movements. Generally, spatial awareness is reduced in hypermobile joints, which has an impact upon the child's balance mechanisms. These factors are also compounded by the fact that the muscles around the joints are not at their optimum strength or stamina, often because joint pain will inhibit muscle action. Therefore, the muscles will become weaker and more unfit at the same time as the child is growing and developing. The muscles are also not used through their full range, as the hypermobile range is often unstable and not used optimally, and so wasting of the muscles occurs. This muscle wasting and weakness is a factor in the poor control of joint movement, particularly in the hypermobile range, and can lead to instability.

Pain

Children's understanding of pain varies depending upon their age, developmental stage, their coping strategies and their experiences. All of this will have an impact upon the degree of pain reported and the importance and significance of the pain experienced.

Consideration needs to be given to other members of the family, not only because they may be anxious on their child's behalf, but also because they may be suffering from the syndrome themselves. A parent's pain problems will have an impact upon the child's experience of pain. The psychological component of pain should always be remembered when dealing with JHS (McGrath 1995).

MANAGEMENT OF THE JOINT HYPERMOBILITY SYNDROME

Medical

Children usually present to their medical practitioner with a history of joint, limb or back pain and generalized fatigue that has a considerable impact upon their day-to-day independent functioning. It is important that when the diagnosis is made, careful clinical assessment has been made to rule out any other condition, with the use of investigations where appropriate. It is also important to avoid unnecessary further invasive tests, and to ensure that the diagnosis and its implications are clearly presented to the family. The family should understand that the condition is relatively benign (compared to juvenile idiopathic arthritis) and that self-management is paramount.

Referral to an allied health professional will prompt an assessment followed by a rehabilitation programme, with a view to self-management by the child and the family.

Therapy management

Subjective assessment

It is important for the therapist to take a full history of the presenting condition, to confirm that other underlying conditions have been ruled out and to establish a clear picture of the nature and severity of the symptoms, their site, frequency and duration. This will enable the treatment plan to be tailor-made to the child's symptoms, and it can also be used as the basis of an outcome measure if recorded accurately. It is useful to use a visual analogue scale for pain if the child is over 7 years old, as it is less subjective, and a 'happy face scale' or 'ouchometer' for younger children.

Children with JHS will often present with painful joints that are most painful in the evenings and after physical activity. The child occasionally complains of stiffness in the mornings, but this rarely lasts for long.

In JHS there is also the issue of developing a downward spiral of recurring acute and chronic pain symptoms, which needs to be broken to avoid a continuation of symptoms (Fig. 4.1). This notion should be explained to the family, and from the assessment the relative proportion and timing of the rest periods and active periods should be defined. It is also important to ascertain when the pain-free times occur: for example always at weekends, requiring the child to recover during the week instead of attending school because of the pain. This should be discussed, as it will ensure that the 'pacing programme' and the return to normal activity are appropriate.

Previous experiences of pain the child has had or personally observed before should be noted, as this may have an impact upon their coping mechanisms. It has been found that children who have experience of another member of the family with chronic pain show that their coping mechanisms are influenced by their observations of others (McGrath 1995). An assessment by a clinical psychologist may be necessary to identify factors that compound the underlying cause of pain in such children and their families (Malleson and Beauchamp 2001).

Objective assessment

When examining a child with JHS it is important to assess the distribution and the degree of hypermobility in the joints involved, as this will influence the treatment programme. The distribution of hypermobility can be scored using one of the scales mentioned previously, but a full assessment of range of movement of every joint is likely to be useful, especially in children with multiple joint symptoms. Some children may have generalized hypermobility, involving most of their joints, whereas others may have a pauciarticular form affecting a small number of peripheral joints.

Once the distribution of joint hypermobility has been assessed, the degree of muscle strength around the joints needs to be examined. It is important for good joint control and stability that the muscles have full strength and normal endurance, especially into the hypermobile range. If this is not the case then arthralgia and muscle fatigue are likely to occur with prolonged activity. The risk of subluxation of joints, although small, is increased when muscle strength and control are less than optimal. Muscle strength can be measured using either the Oxford Scale, the expanded 11-point scale (0–10, Kendall et al. 1993), or by using myometry.

Children with JHS are usually generally unfit and have very poor stamina. This also needs to be addressed in a rehabilitation programme. Stamina is often assessed subjectively, but the '6-minute walk test' (Boardman et al. 2000, Garofano and Barst 1999, Hamilton and Haennel 2000, King et al. 2000, Nixon et al. 1996, Pankoff et al. 2000) is a better objective measure. This test requires the subject to walk as fast and as far as

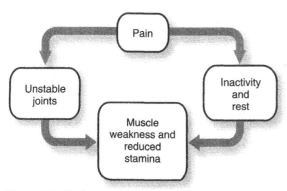

Figure 4.1 Vicious cycle of pain

he or she can in 6 minutes. The distance walked and the time taken (if he or she is unable to manage the 6 minutes) are then recorded.

As with any musculoskeletal assessment, it is important to observe the posture and gait of the child and to watch for any abnormalities that might be due to the hypermobility. The most common posture and gait disturbances are:

- Hyperlordosis of the lumbar spine;
- Increased kyphosis in the thoracic spine;
- Weakness around the hips causing a Trendelenburg sign;
- Hyperextension of the knees in the weight-bearing position;
- Pronated/flat feet.

Once the child has been fully assessed, the specific problems identified can be included in an individualized rehabilitation programme.

Diminished balance and poor proprioception are often an issue for children with JHS (Hall et al. 1995, Mallik et al. 1994), and these also need to be assessed at the initial stage. Asking the child to stand on one leg and observing his or her balance can give a simple measure, which is then progressed further by asking him or her to close his or her eyes at the same time. Removing the visual input will assess proprioception more specifically. A more in-depth assessment can be included by isolating each joint and assessing spatial awareness without the visual input, i.e. asking the child to identify the direction of movement of a joint while keeping his or her eyes shut.

Aims of treatment

It is a common misconception that the purpose of treatment is to reduce the range of mobility of the joints. The real purpose of the rehabilitation programme, however, is to improve the stability and control of the joint while maintaining the full normal hypermobile range of movement. Therefore the aims of treatment are:

- To increase the strength of the muscles, especially into the hypermobile range;
- To improve the stamina of the muscles;

- To improve the general fitness of the child;
- To re-educate gait to avoid/correct any abnormalities in the biomechanics;
- To return to normal activities and functioning;
- To educate the child and family to enable them to manage the condition with minimal reliance on medication.

These aims work together to ensure that the child has more stable joints, protected by strong, fit muscles enabling him or her to manage his or her symptoms independently at home with the minimum of external support, i.e. splints, professional support etc.

TREATMENT METHODS

Joint stability and muscle strength

The inherent stability of a joint is determined by the efficiency or integrity of the musculoskeletal system (muscle, tendon, capsule, ligament and articular surfaces) and the neural control systems (motor and sensory). As discussed previously, one hypothesis suggests that JHS may be a result of abnormal collagen fibres resulting in ligamentous insufficiency. The soft-tissue microtrauma caused by this insufficiency is one accepted explanation for the joint and muscle pains (Gedalia and Brewer 1993). It follows, then, that improving dynamic muscle control in order to compensate for the ligamentous insufficiency should minimize the trauma (Kerr et al. 2000).

It is commonly recognized that children respond well to a muscle-strengthening programme, and although they may not improve their muscle bulk, they do improve strength and neuromuscular coordination, thereby making the muscles more effective (Barton and Bird 1996, Biro et al. 1983, Finsterbush and Pogrund 1982). In general it appears clear that the treatment of choice for children with JHS is a muscle-strengthening programme working through their full range of movement, including the hypermobile range (Kerr et al. 2000, Russek 1999, 2000).

When devising an exercise programme, all aspects of muscle function need to be considered, including isometric, isotonic, concentric and eccentric strength, stamina and general function. It is ideal to start with a programme that isolates each muscle group individually, and includes all aspects of its function. It is also important to ensure that all muscle groups around the joint are strengthened equally, i.e. for the knee both quadriceps and hamstrings, in order to ensure physiological balance. It is often useful, especially if the child is experiencing significant pain, to start with some static exercises in the hypermobile range before progressing to dynamic and then resisted work (Borms 1986). These should also be progressed from non-weight-bearing work to weight-bearing work.

Stamina or endurance training is also very important for the muscles, as it is extremely important to have not only strong muscles, but muscles that will not fatigue easily. Therefore, an exercise regimen of high repetitions and low weights is used, which is usually achievable and sustainable in a self-management home exercise programme.

Splinting of hypermobile joints is rarely recommended as this is likely to exacerbate ineffective muscle use, causing them to become weaker still and more prone to injury. In addition it can, in effect, inhibit the rehabilitation programme and add to the impression that there is a more serious medical disorder requiring therapy to be provided, rather than solely from the parents and child's own home management. However, the use of limited types of support, or devices such as pen grips, can be a good adjunct to a hand muscle-strengthening programme. They reduce the force required to sustain the gripping of a pen, thereby reducing the pain and fatigue experienced in the fingers and wrists during school work, for example.

Children with JHS often present with very pronated, flat feet as a result of their hypermobility, which can contribute to lower limb symptoms. This problem will often respond very well to the use of orthotics in the shoes, which take the form of heel cups or arch supports that support and control the subtalar joint and medial arch, helping to improve foot position. Although it can be argued that this may encourage weaker foot muscles, in practice the benefits of correcting the biomechanics of the foot have such a positive effect on the whole gait pattern that it is a preferred form of treatment (Agnew 1997). In many cases correcting the biomechanics of the feet significantly reduces the abnormal forces throughout the other joints, thereby reducing the pain (such as an anterior knee pain) experienced.

Gait re-education

A combination of hypermobile joints, reduced proprioception, weak muscles and reduced stamina can profoundly affect the gait of a child with JHS. To correct this, the causes of the abnormalities need to be identified and treated separately. However, it is important that the child recognizes the abnormalities in his or her gait and is taught how to correct them. Positive feedback, using video recording and mirrors, can aid this process.

Hand function

Finger joint laxity is one of the most common features of hypermobility in the upper limbs, and as a result hand function is often impaired. This is seen particularly in schoolchildren, where prolonged writing tasks become necessary. In some children it is important to include an exercise programme specifically for the fingers and wrists to improve pain-free function and to protect the joints. This can include exercises with putty, micro-theraband or wax, as well as assessing the posture during the performance of tasks and working on any ineffectiveness. The use of pen grips or fat pens and regular periods of rest may help with sloppy writing, but the provision of splints should be avoided. Occupational therapy assessment of writing function is often very useful to help to correct abnormal positions of fingers, hand and general posture, as well as provide ideas to correct this, such as the provision of a sloping writing board. It is also important to consider the ergonomics of the chairs and tables and other school equipment being used to ensure the optimum posture is achieved.

Functional tasks

Children with JHS often adapt to their hypermobility by altering the mechanics of how they function, leading to increased pain, pain in other locations, and an increase in the fatigue suffered. It is therefore important to work on specific functional activities and to develop with the child energy-saving, biomechanically correct, safe and pain-free ways of performing these activities. Movements involved in these activities can be practised and included in the rehabilitation programme, i.e. step-ups on a stair, repeated sitting to stand from a chair, etc.

Balance

Given that proprioception and balance are often reduced in children with JHS, techniques related to these problems should be incorporated into the programme. This can easily be done by encouraging the child to practise standing on one leg, without shoes and socks on, while maintaining a good posture. It is important to ensure the child is made aware of controlling knee hyperextension, if present. This exercise can be progressed by using a balance (wobble) board. The use of rhythmic stabilizations is also a useful method to improve postural stability, both globally and specifically. Weight-bearing exercises are essential and should be given for both upper limbs (prone kneeling etc.) and lower limbs.

General fitness

Children with JHS will often have been very sedentary because of their pain, and are usually generally unfit. It is therefore important to incorporate some aerobic fitness work into the rehabilitation programme. Care needs to be taken early on, when they still have suboptimal muscle strength, to ensure that the fitness aspect of the programme is of low impact so that joint symptoms are not increased and the child and family do not lose faith in the programme. The authors have frequently seen resistance by the child and family to physiotherapy interventions, as they have often experienced previous attempts that have increased their pain. This is usually a result of starting the programme too vigorously, progressing too fast, and/or poor compliance.

Swimming is a highly desirable method of exercise as it is usually 'low stress' for the joints and is a good aerobic activity. It is preferable that a normal swimming pool is used for ongoing management, as hydrotherapy pools are too hot for distance swimming.

Bicycling is also very good for aerobic work and, similarly, does not overstress the other joints. However, as soon as strength is improving, normal aerobic and sporting activities can be included, providing they form part of the pacing programme.

Hydrotherapy

Hydrotherapy can be a very beneficial adjunct to the treatment of JHS. The heat will provide pain relief and help to reduce any muscle spasm, and the effects of buoyancy will support the joints, allowing strengthening exercises to be performed. This is often very useful at the beginning of the treatment programme, when pain and stiffness are often significant. Hydrotherapy provides many opportunities to work on the strength of specific muscles and stamina, as well as postural stability.

Pain relief

It is important for the child and family to understand that the pain is due to the hypermobility and associated musculoskeletal insufficiencies, and not to any other rheumatological condition. The family often needs to be reassured that the pain will ease, but only when the muscles are strong and fit and are protecting the joints more fully, and when the child is functioning normally both biomechanically and generally (i.e. walking correctly and attending school fully, etc.). It is often found that the pain is slow to improve, and this should be emphasized at the start of the programme. Children and parents are often counselled that rehabilitation will be prolonged. A child who has had 18 months of pain and disability may take a similar length of time before returning to full pain-free independent function. It is difficult to quantify the degree of pain that is acceptable within the rehabilitation programme, but we expect the pain to be moderate to mild in degree. It may be expected to recur on-and-off over the years, often becoming worse if the child becomes unfit. It is important for the child and family to realize that the pain of hypermobility does not signify damage or illness, but is an indicator of poor joint control and therefore benign and manageable.

Other methods of pain relief may be of use, such as hot or cold packs on specific joints. Transcutaneous nerve stimulation (TENS) may also have a role to play in this aspect, but it must be seen only as a supportive treatment and not a solution, and must not replace the rehabilitation programme. Relaxation and distraction techniques can be used to help the child or young person manage their pain. This is often useful at night if they have difficulty sleeping because of the pain and discomfort. It can also be used in many other situations, for example at school during breaks, to ensure that they are able to manage the rest of the day. Massage may also be a very effective way of easing any pain, especially if it is due to muscle spasm.

Formal psychological input may be required, but in the authors' experience this is usually necessary in less than 10% of cases. Psychological support by healthcare providers for hypermobile patients with pain is uniformly beneficial and provided for most patients in our hospital. This includes listening carefully to their pain story and providing pain management strategies for them to practise.

Pacing

Pacing is an extremely important part of the rehabilitation of a child with JHS.

It is very often the case that the child will report that they will play football, go swimming, go out with their friends and dance at the weekend. They are then very sore on Monday and are unable to attend school; however, by the weekend they have recovered enough to be able to do many activities again, and the cycle continues. This causes a constant 'peaking and troughing' of symptoms and causes a major disruption to life. Eventually this may form part of a 'school refusal' pattern.

Pacing activities are taught to stop this behaviour completely and help them build up again slowly. Therefore specific tasks are set for each day, which are achievable without giving rise to a significant increase in symptoms. These tasks must be completed, no more and no less, whether it is a good or a bad day. For this programme to work effectively everyone involved in the care of the child, such as the child, parents, school and therapist, should be included in planning the pacing. A written agreement may be used to facilitate progression and to ensure that the programme is developed between the therapist and the family. It is also useful to develop a 'back-up' plan if problems arise, to prevent the original problems from developing again or, if they do, to bring them more rapidly under control. Further guidance on pacing is given in Chapter 10.

Psychology

In some cases where pain and loss of independent function are profound, it is important to include the clinical psychologist in the management team. They will be able to help develop pain management skills for the child, as well as generally help the family cope with the condition and to understand its impact on the whole family. Many families find this support invaluable and are able to change many unhelpful coping strategies into helpful ones, leaving behind the 'chronic pain cycle' that may have developed in the preceding phase.

Case study

RJ is a 12-year-old girl who at the age of 10 presented with pains in her ankles. Initially the ankles became painful in the evenings of the day she had been doing PE at school. She stopped doing PE for a while and, as the pain did not improve, she rested at home for a week. When she returned to school the pains became worse and spread to her knees and hips, and she also developed pain in her fingers. She found that the pain was worse in the evenings after school.

Developmentally RJ was slow to crawl and to walk, and was often falling over. She bruised easily and suffered pain in her legs at night.

RJ's mother also suffered from growing pains as a child; she had trained as a dancer until she was 21, and was still very mobile.

The GP, who could find no evidence of any swelling of the joints, suggested paracetamol and recommended staying at school.

Over the next 6 months RJ was able to go to school less and less because of the pain, but found that she was able to play with her friends and go out shopping at weekends, although by Monday she was too sore for school. The GP then referred her to a paediatrician, who was able to exclude any pathology and diagnosed joint hypermobility syndrome. She was then referred to a paediatric physiotherapist.

At the physiotherapy assessment RJ was still complaining of pain in her hands, wrists, hips, knees and ankles. The pain was reasonably constant and prevented her from going to school; however, she tried very hard at the weekend and was able to go out and play with her friends and spend the day shopping with them. They also often went bowling or ice-skating in the evenings. Her school had been very supportive and had been sending work home, but RJ was only able to write for 10 minutes before her hands became painful.

On examination all joints were hypermobile and lax, and she scored 9/9 on the Beighton score. She also had considerable muscle weakness, both proximally and distally, averaging 3+/5 (Oxford Scale). Her balance was reduced and she had pronated, flat feet.

An outpatient treatment plan was designed, starting with a specific problem list:
1. Pain in fingers, wrists, hips, knees and ankles
2. Global muscle weakness
3. Poor balance
4. Abnormal posture
5. Poor school attendance
6. Joint hypermobility
7. Reduced general stamina and fitness.

Aims of treatment
1. Educate RJ and her family about JHS and the importance of a paced musculoskeletal self-management approach.
2. Teach RJ how to manage her pain to enable her to function independently.
3. Increase muscle strength, stamina and fitness throughout the body.
4. Improve general balance and stability.
5. Improve posture.
6. Develop a graduated return to school.

Ultimate goals
1. To achieve full attendance at school and participation in all activities.
2. To gain a full understanding of hypermobility and the principles of self-management.
3. To feel in control of her pain.

Methods of treatment
Initially a home exercise programme was developed which included exercises to improve balance, stability and the strength of lower and upper limb muscles. The exercises were all started with 10 repetitions and gradually progressed to 30. Once 30 repetitions could be achieved correctly the programme was progressed further by the addition of weights, initially 1 lb increasing to a maximum of 3 lb.

Pacing of activities was discussed at length with RJ and her family, and a meeting was arranged at her school. At this meeting a gradual return to full function was planned. During week 1 it was agreed that she would attend school for 1 hour a day, perform her exercise programme once a day, participate in one fun activity, such as swimming for 30 minutes, and take part in gentle activities around the home. At the weekend 1 hour of schoolwork was substituted for the 1 hour at school.

In week 2 she increased her attendance at school to half a day and continued her exercise programme once a day, a fun activity for 30 minutes, and at the weekend she did 1 hour of schoolwork and 2 hours of fun activity.

This was continued until RJ achieved full attendance at school and was able to participate fully in weekend activities as well.

Physiotherapy appointments were arranged initially twice weekly for the first 4 weeks, and then reduced to once weekly for a further 4 weeks and then twice monthly for 2 months. She was then given a review appointment every 3 months, with the option of an earlier appointment if necessary. After three review appointments RJ was discharged.

Initially physiotherapy consisted of teaching the home exercise programme, relaxation techniques, explaining the condition and discussing the treatment plan. During subsequent sessions the home exercise programme was progressed, and included exercising on a balance board, working on proximal stability and strength using a Swiss ball and weight-bearing exercises, increasing stamina using a static bicycle, including functional activities such as step-ups and intrinsic foot muscle exercises.

Insoles were also provided to correct the position of the feet and thereby improve the biomechanics of the lower limbs.

Outcome
After 1 month of treatment RJ was back at school full time and was able to join in several activities at the weekend; however, she still had some pain. At 6 months RJ was completely independent and was able to do all activities, but she still had some pain in her fingers, wrists and ankles. At 1 year RJ was discharged from treatment and complained of only very occasional pain that she could manage by maintaining her exercise programme 3–4 times weekly with 30 repeats and a 3 lb weight.

CONCLUSION

Joint hypermobility syndrome can present in many young people. If untreated or undiagnosed it can result in the development of a 'chronic pain cycle' and a high level of disability. This requires an intensive but paced musculoskeletal rehabilitation programme to manage the symptoms effectively. It is vital that the child and family are clear in their understanding of the condition, and that a self–management programme is the most appropriate long-term treatment approach.

REFERENCES

Acasuso-Diaz, M. and Collantes-Estevez, E. (1998) Joint hypermobility in patients with fibromyalgia syndrome. *Arthritis Care and Research*, **11**, 39–42.

Agnew, P. (1997) Evaluation of the child with ligamentous laxity. *Clinics in Podiatry Medicine and Surgery*, **14**, 117–30.

Al-Rawi, Z. and Nessan, A.H. (1997) Joint hypermobility in patients with chondromalacia patellae. *British Journal of Rheumatology*, **36**, 1324–7.

Arroyo, I.L., Brewer, E.J. and Giannini, E.H. (1988) Arthritis/arthralgia and hypermobility of the joints in schoolchildren. *Journal of Rheumatology*, **15**, 978–80.

Augustsson, J. and Thomee, R. (2000) Ability of closed and open kinetic chain tests of muscular strength to assess functional performance. *Scandinavian Journal of Medical Science Sports*, **10**, 164–8.

Barton, L.M. and Bird, H.A. (1996) Improving pain by the stabilization of hyperlax joints. *Journal of Orthopaedic Rheumatology*, **9**, 46–51.

Beighton, P., de Paepe, A. and Danks, D. (1988) International nosology of heritable disorders of connective tissue, Berlin. *American Journal of Medical Genetics*, **29**, 581–94.

Beighton, P., Solomon, L. and Soskolne, C.L. (1973) Articular mobility in an African population. *Annals of the Rheumatic Diseases*, **32**, 413–18.

Beighton, P.H. and Horan, F.T. (1970) Dominant inheritance in familial generalised articular hypermobility. *Journal of Bone and Joint Surgery [British]*, **52**, 145–7.

Bensahel, H., Souchet, P., Pennecot, G. and Mazda, K. (2000) The unstable patella in children. *Journal of Pediatric Orthopedics*, **9**, 265–70.

Bird, H.A., Brodie, D.A. and Wright, V. (1979) Quantification of joint laxity. *Rheumatology and Rehabilitation*, **18**, 161–6.

Bird, H.A., Tribe, C.R. and Bacon, P.A. (1978) Joint hypermobility leading to osteoarthrosis and chondrocalcinosis. *Annals of the Rheumatic Diseases*, **37**, 203–11.

Biro, F., Gewanter, H.L. and Baum, J. (1983) The hypermobility syndrome. *Pediatrics*, **72**, 701–6.

Birrell, F.N., Adebajo, A.O., Hazleman, B.L. and Silman, A. J. (1994) High prevalence of joint laxity in West Africans. *British Journal of Rheumatology*, **33**, 56–9.

Boardman, D.L., Dorey, F., Thomas, B.J. and Lieberman, J.R. (2000) The accuracy of assessing total hip arthroplasty outcomes: a prospective correlation study of walking ability and 2 validated measurement devices. *Journal of Arthroplasty*, **15**, 200–4.

Borms, J. (1986) The child and exercise: an overview. *Journal of Sports Science*, **4**, 3–20.

Bridges, A.J., Smith, E. and Reid, J. (1992) Joint hypermobility in adults referred to rheumatology clinics. *Annals of the Rheumatic Diseases*, **51**, 793–6.

Buckingham, R.B., Braun, T., Harinstein, D.A. et al. (1991) Temporomandibular joint dysfunction syndrome: a close association with systemic joint laxity (the hypermobile joint syndrome). *Oral Surgery, Oral Medicine, Oral Pathology*, **72**, 514–19.

Bulbena, A., Duro, J.C., Porta, M. et al. (1992) Clinical assessment of hypermobility of joints: assembling criteria. *Journal of Rheumatology*, **19**, 115–22.

Bulbena, A., Duro, J.C., Porta, M. et al. (1993) Anxiety disorders in the joint hypermobility syndrome. *Psychiatry Research*, **46**, 59–68.

Buskila, D., Neumann, L., Hershman, E. et al. (1995) Fibromyalgia syndrome in children – an outcome study. *Journal of Rheumatology*, **22**, 525–8.

Carter, C. and Wilkinson, J. (1964) Persistent joint laxity and congenital dislocation of the hip. *Journal of Bone and Joint Surgery [British]*, **46**, 40–5.

Cheng, J.C., Chan, P.S. and Hui, P.W. (1991) Joint laxity in children. *Journal of Pediatric Orthopedics*, **11**, 752–6.

Child, A.H. (1986) Joint hypermobility syndrome: inherited disorder of collagen synthesis. *Journal of Rheumatology*, **13**, 239–43.

Conti, P.C., Miranda, J.E. and Araujo, C.R. (2000) Relationship between systemic joint laxity, TMJ hypertranslation, and intra-articular disorders. *Journal of Craniomandibular Practice*, **18**, 192–7.

Davidovitch, M., Tirosh, E. and Tal, Y. (1994) The relationship between joint hypermobility and neurodevelopmental attributes in elementary school children. *Journal of Child Neurology*, **9**, 417–19.

Decoster, L.C., Vailas, J.C., Lindsay, R.H. and Williams, G. R. (1997) Prevalence and features of joint hypermobility among adolescent athletes. *Archive of Pediatric and Adolescent Medicine*, **151**, 989–92.

Dolan, A.L., Arden, N.K., Grahame, R. and Spector, T.D. (1998) Assessment of bone in Ehlers–Danlos syndrome by ultrasound and densitometry. *Annals of the Rheumatic Diseases*, **57**, 630–3.

El-Garf, A.K., Mahmoud, G.A. and Mahgoub, E.H. (1998) Hypermobility among Egyptian children: prevalence and features. *Journal of Rheumatology*, **25**, 1003–5.

El-Shahaly, H.A. and El-Sherif, A.K. (1991) Is the benign joint hypermobility syndrome benign? *Clinical Rheumatology*, **10**, 302–7.

Engelbert, R.H., Beemer, F.A., van Der, G.Y. and Helders, P.J. (1999) Osteogenesis imperfecta in childhood: impairment and disability – a follow-up study. *Archives of Physical and Medical Rehabilitation*, **80**, 896–903.

Engelbert, R.H., Gerver, W.J., Breslau-Siderius, L.J. et al. (1998) Spinal complications in osteogenesis imperfecta: 47 patients 1–16 years of age. *Acta Orthopedica Scandinavica*, **69**, 283–6.

Finsterbush, A. and Pogrund, H. (1982) The hypermobility syndrome. Musculoskeletal complaints in 100 consecutive cases of generalized joint hypermobility. *Clinical Orthopedics*, **168**, 124–7.

Forleo, L.H., Hilario, M.O., Peixoto, A.L. et al. (1993). Articular hypermobility in school children in Sao Paulo, Brazil. *Journal of Rheumatology*, **20**, 916–17.

Francis, H., March, L., Terenty, T. and Webb, J. (1987) Benign joint hypermobility with neuropathy: documentation and mechanism of tarsal tunnel syndrome. *Journal of Rheumatology*, **14**, 577–81.

Garofano, R.P. and Barst, R.J. (1999) Exercise testing in children with primary pulmonary hypertension. *Pediatric Cardiology*, **20**, 61–4.

Gedalia, A. and Brewer, E.J. (1993) Joint hypermobility in pediatric practice – a review. *Journal of Rheumatology*, **20**, 371–4.

Gedalia, A., Garcia, C.O., Molina, J.F. et al. (2000) Fibromyalgia syndrome: experience in a pediatric rheumatology clinic. *Clinical and Experimental Rheumatology*, **18**, 415–19.

Gedalia, A., Person, D.A., Brewer, E.J. and Giannini, E.H. (1985) Hypermobility of the joints in juvenile episodic arthritis/arthralgia. *Journal of Pediatrics*, **107**, 873–6.

Gedalia, A. and Press, J. (1998) Joint hypermobility and musculoskeletal pain. *Journal of Rheumatology*, **25**, 1031–2.

Gedalia, A., Press, J., Klein, M. and Buskila, D. (1993) Joint hypermobility and fibromyalgia in schoolchildren. *Annals of the Rheumatic Diseases*, **52**, 494–6.

Goldman, J.A. (1991) Hypermobility and deconditioning: important links to fibromyalgia/fibrositis. *Southern Medical Journal*, **84**, 1192–6.

Grahame, R. (1999) Joint hypermobility and genetic collagen disorders: are they related? *Archives of Disease in Childhood*, **80**, 188–91.

Grahame, R. (2000) Hypermobility – not a circus act. *International Journal of Clinical Practice*, **54**, 314–15.

Grahame, R., Bird, H.A., Child, A. et al. (2000) The revised (Brighton 1998) criteria for the diagnosis of benign joint hypermobility syndrome (BJHS). *Journal of Rheumatology*, **27**, 1777–9.

Grahame, R., Edwards, J.C., Pitcher, D. et al. (1981) A clinical and echocardiographic study of patients with the hypermobility syndrome. *Annals of the Rheumatic Diseases*, **40**, 541–6.

Grahame, R. and Pyeritz, R.E. (1995) The Marfan syndrome: joint and skin manifestations are prevalent and correlated. *British Journal of Rheumatology*, **34**, 126–31.

Gulan, G., Matovinovic, D., Nemec, B. et al. (2000) Femoral neck anteversion: values, development, measurement, common problems. *Collegium Antropologicum*, **24**, 521–7.

Hagroo, G.A., Zaki, H.M., Choudhary, M.T. and Hussain, A. (1995) Pulled elbow – not the effect of hypermobility of joints. *Injury*, **26**, 687–90.

Hall, M.G., Ferrell, W.R., Sturrock, R.D. et al. (1995) The effect of the hypermobility syndrome on knee joint proprioception. *British Journal of Rheumatology*, **34**, 121–5.

Hamilton, D.M. and Haennel, R.G. (2000) Validity and reliability of the 6-minute walk test in a cardiac rehabilitation population. *Journal of Cardiopulmonary Rehabilitation*, **20**, 156–64.

Hamilton, P.R. and Broughton, N.S. (1998) Traumatic hip dislocation in childhood. *Journal of Pediatric Orthopedics*, **18**, 691–4.

Handler, C.E., Child, A., Light, N.D. and Dorrance, D.E. (1985) Mitral valve prolapse, aortic compliance, and skin collagen in joint hypermobility syndrome. *British Heart Journal*, **54**, 501–8.

Henney, A.M., Brotherton, D.H., Child, A.H. et al. (1992) Segregation analysis of collagen genes in two families with joint hypermobility syndrome. *British Journal of Rheumatology*, **31**, 169–74.

Horton, W.A., Collins, D.L., DeSmet, A.A. et al. (1980) Familial joint instability syndrome. *American Journal of Medical Genetics*, **6**, 221–8.

Howell, D.W. (1984) Musculoskeletal profile and incidence of musculoskeletal injuries in lightweight women rowers. *American Journal of Sports Medicine*, **12**, 278–82.

Hudson, N., Fitzcharles, M.A., Cohen, M. et al. (1998) The association of soft-tissue rheumatism and hypermobility. *British Journal of Rheumatology*, **37**, 382–6.

Hudson, N., Starr, M.R., Esdaile, J. M. and Fitzcharles, M.A. (1995) Diagnostic associations with hypermobility in rheumatology patients. *British Journal of Rheumatology*, **34**, 1157–61.

Jaffe, M., Tirosh, E., Cohen, A. and Taub, Y. (1988) Joint mobility and motor development. *Archives of Disease in Childhood*, **63**, 159–61.

Jessee, E.F., Owen, D.S. Jr and Sagar, K.B. (1980) The benign hypermobile joint syndrome. *Arthritis and Rheumatism*, **23**, 1053–5.

Kendall, F.P., McCreary, E.K. and Provance, P.G. (1993) *Muscles: Testing and Function*, 4th edn. Williams and Wilkins.

Kerr, A., Macmillan, C.E., Uttley, W.S. and Luqmani, R.A. (2000) Physiotherapy for children with hypermobility syndrome. *Physiotherapy*, **86**, 313–17.

Khan, F.A. and Pedlar, J. (1996) Generalized joint hypermobility as a factor in clicking of the temporomandibular joint. *International Journal of Oral and Maxillofacial Surgery*, **25**, 101–4.

King, M.B., Judge, J.O., Whipple, R. and Wolfson, L. (2000) Reliability and responsiveness of two physical performance measures examined in the context of a functional training intervention. *Physical Therapy*, **80**, 8–16.

Kirk, J.A., Ansell, B.M. and Bywaters, E.G. (1967) The hypermobility syndrome. Musculoskeletal complaints associated with generalized joint hypermobility. *Annals of the Rheumatic Diseases*, **26**, 419–25.

Lannoo, E., De Paepe, A., Leroy, B. and Thiery, E. (1996) Neuropsychological aspects of Marfan syndrome. *Clinical Genetics*, **49**, 65–9.

Larsson, L. G., Baum, J. and Mudholkar, G. S. (1987) Hypermobility: features and differential incidence between the sexes. *Arthritis and Rheumatism*, **30**, 1426–30.

Larsson, L.G., Baum, J., Mudholkar, G.S. and Kollia, G.D. (1993) Benefits and disadvantages of joint hypermobility among musicians. *New England Journal of Medicine*, **329**, 1079–82.

Larsson, L.G., Mudholkar, G.S., Baum, J. and Srivastava, D.K. (1995) Benefits and liabilities of hypermobility in the back pain disorders of industrial workers. *Journal of Internal Medicine*, **238**, 461–7.

Lewkonia, R.M. and Ansell, B.M. (1983) Articular hypermobility simulating chronic rheumatic disease. *Archives of Disease in Childhood*, **58**, 988–92.

Malleson, P.N. and Beauchamp, R.D. (2001) Rheumatology: 16. Diagnosing musculoskeletal pain in children. *Canadian Medical Association Journal*, **165**, 183–8.

Mallik, A.K., Ferrell, W.R., McDonald, A.G. and Sturrock, R. D. (1994) Impaired proprioceptive acuity at the proximal interphalangeal joint in patients with the hypermobility syndrome. *British Journal of Rheumatology*, **33**, 631–7.

McGrath, P.J. (1995) Annotation: aspects of pain in children and adolescents. *Journal of Child Psychology and Psychiatry*, **36**, 717–30.

Mishra, M.B., Ryan, P., Atkinson, P. et al. (1996) Extra-articular features of benign joint hypermobility syndrome. *British Journal of Rheumatology*, **35**, 861–6.

Moreira, A. and Wilson, J. (1992) Non-progressive paraparesis in children with congenital ligamentous laxity. *Neuropediatrics*, **23**, 49–52.

Murray, K.J. and Woo, P. (2001) Benign joint hypermobility in childhood. *Rheumatology*, **40**, 489–91.

Nixon, P.A., Joswiak, M.L. and Fricker, F.J. (1996) A six-minute walk test for assessing exercise tolerance in severely ill children. *Journal of Pediatrics*, **129**, 362–6.

Pankoff, B., Overend, T., Lucy, D. and White, K. (2000) Validity and responsiveness of the 6 minute walk test for people with fibromyalgia. *Journal of Rheumatology*, **27**, 2666–70.

Pepin, M., Schwarze, U., Superti-Furga, A. and Byers, P. H. (2000) Clinical and genetic features of Ehlers–Danlos syndrome type IV, the vascular type. *New England Journal of Medicine*, **342**, 673–80.

Perrini, F., Tallents, R.H., Katzberg, R.W. et al. (1997) Generalized joint laxity and temporomandibular disorders. *Journal of Orofacial Pain*, **11**, 215–21.

Prockop, D.J. and Kivirikko, K.I. (1995) Collagens: molecular biology, diseases, and potentials for therapy. *Annual Review of Biochemistry*, **64**, 403–34.

Pyeritz, R.E. (2000) Ehlers–Danlos syndrome. *New England Journal of Medicine*, **342**, 730–2.

Qvindesland, A. and Jonsson, H. (1999) Articular hypermobility in Icelandic 12-year-olds. *Rheumatology* (Oxford), **38**, 1014–16.

Raff, M.L. and Byers, P.H. (1996) Joint hypermobility syndromes. *Current Opinion in Rheumatology*, **8**, 459–66.

Rikken-Bultman, D.G., Wellink, L. and van Dongen, P.W. (1997) Hypermobility in two Dutch school populations. *European Journal of Obstetrics, Gynecology and Reproductive Biology*, **73**, 189–92.

Runow, A. (1983) The dislocating patella. Etiology and prognosis in relation to generalized joint laxity and anatomy of the patellar articulation. *Acta Orthopedica Scandinavica*, **201** Suppl., 1–53.

Russek, L.N. (1999) Hypermobility syndrome. *Physical Therapy*, **79**, 591–9.

Russek, L.N. (2000) Examination and treatment of a patient with hypermobility syndrome. *Physical Therapy*, **80**, 386–98.

Scharf, Y. and Nahir, A.M. (1982) Case report: hypermobility syndrome mimicking juvenile chronic arthritis. *Rheumatology and Rehabilitation*, **21**, 78–80.

Seow, C.C., Chow, P.K. and Khong, K.S. (1999) A study of joint mobility in a normal population. *Annals of the Academy of Medicine of Singapore*, **28**, 231–6.

Silverman, S., Constine, L., Harvey, W. and Grahame, R. (1975) Survey of joint mobility and in vivo skin elasticity in London schoolchildren. *Annals of the Rheumatic Diseases*, **34**, 177–80.

Snead, M.P. and Yates, J.R. (1999) Clinical and molecular genetics of Stickler syndrome. *Journal of Medical Genetics*, **36**, 353–9.

Stanitski, C.L. (1995) Articular hypermobility and chondral injury in patients with acute patellar dislocation. *American Journal of Sports Medicine*, **23**, 146–50.

Tirosh, E., Jaffe, M., Marmur, R. et al. (1991) Prognosis of motor development and joint hypermobility. *Archives of Disease in Childhood*, **66**, 931–3.

Visser, M., Deeg, D.J., Lips, P. et al. (2000) Skeletal muscle mass and muscle strength in relation to lower-extremity performance in older men and women. *Journal of the American Geriatrics Society*, **48**, 381–6.

Vougiouka, O., Moustaki, M. and Tsanaktsi, M. (2000) Benign hypermobility syndrome in Greek schoolchildren. *European Journal of Pediatrics*, **159**, 628.

Wenger, D.R. and Frick, S.L. (1999) Early surgical correction of residual hip dysplasia: the San Diego Children's Hospital approach. *Acta Orthopedica Belgica*, **65**, 277–87.

Winocur, E., Gavish, A., Halachmi, M. et al. (2000) Generalized joint laxity and its relation with oral habits and temporomandibular disorders in adolescent girls. *Journal of Oral Rehabilitation*, **27**, 614–22.

5

Management of the hypermobile adolescent

Alison Middleditch

Aims

1. To review the normal developmental changes that occur during adolescence and consider their impact on adolescents with hypermobility
2. To discuss the musculoskeletal problems that often affect hypermobile adolescents
3. To discuss psychosocial issues, the role of exercise and sport, and management of the hypermobile adolescent

---

INTRODUCTION

Hypermobility in adolescence is complicated by additional problems related to the individual's physical maturity and sociological development. The physical, physiological and psychological changes that occur during adolescence have a bearing on the diagnosis and management of joint hypermobility.

Joint laxity is usually greatest at birth, decreases during childhood, and continues to reduce during adolescence and adult life. The tightness or relative laxity of a ligament is an important element in governing the available joint range of an individual. Laxity of ligaments is determined by an individual's genetic make-up, and the genes that encode collagen, elastin and fibrillin are important in influencing joint flexibility. A number of other factors have an impact on range of joint movement, such as the shape of the joint surfaces, muscle length, and the mobility of the neural structures. These factors continue to change throughout the adolescent growth period, thereby affecting the extent of range of movement in both those who have hypermobility and those with 'normal tissues'. Although an adolescent may be unaware that they are hypermobile, they may believe themselves to be 'double-jointed' and use their excessive range of movement to perform 'tricks'. The hypermobile condition may only become apparent if an injury occurs or the individual develops pain or other problems.

Hypermobility may be inherited or acquired, and joint mobility can be increased with training. Those with 'normal tissues' can increase range of movement by stretching, and this is typically seen in ballet dancers and gymnasts. It is probable that individuals who have joints of average flexibility have better protection from injury by their 'normal tissues', and those who have developed a hypermobile range from specific training enhance the stability of their joints through good muscle strength and control. Although an increase in joint laxity is considered an advantage for some sports and activities, the generally weaker tissue of a hypermobile individual means that they are more susceptible to injury (Grahame and Jenkins 1972). The joints are frequently less stable and vulnerable to subluxation or dislocation. A feature of hypermobile tissues is that they are less resilient, so that muscle tears and tendon–osseous attachment lesions (e.g. epicondylitis and plantar fasciitis) occur with greater ease (Grahame 1999).

Children with hypermobility are often attracted to physical activities such as gymnastics and ballet. Good muscle tone, particularly of the deep postural muscles, helps to protect against injury and improves joint stability. Hypermobile ballet dancers have a higher incidence of injuries than non-hypermobile dancers (Klemp et al. 1984) and these injuries commonly affect the feet, knees and lower back. Flexible joints can have a tendency to instability, and without adequate muscular support movements such as handstands and balancing on one leg can be more difficult. Hyperlaxity of the tarsal and first tarsometatarsal joints can prevent a ballet dancer from dancing *en pointe* (Beighton et al. 1989a).

Children and adolescents are susceptible to the same acute and overuse sporting injuries as adults (Thein 1996), and the incidence of injury is greater in adolescents than in children (Zaricznyj et al. 1980, Apple 1985). An understanding of normal development and the physical, physiological and psychological changes that occur during adolescence is particularly important when dealing with a hypermobile teenager who has a sporting injury.

Hypermobility is also considered to be an advantage for musicians. The increased flexibility improves dexterity and allows a greater span of the fingers. Larsson et al. (1993) found that violinists, flautists and pianists who have lax finger joints suffer less pain than those who have relatively stiffer joints. Musicians require many of the same characteristics as athletes: they need excellent coordination, good muscle strength and endurance. Musicians are susceptible to the same acute and overuse injuries as athletes, and a young musician who has hypermobility will benefit from incorporating warm-up, cool-down and strengthening exercises into their practise sessions. A review of the adolescent hypermobiles who attended our clinic over a 2-year period showed that about 20% presented with problems related to playing an instrument (unpublished data).

ONSET OF SYMPTOMS

Approximately 7–10% of the school-aged population has loose joints and occasional pain in joints and muscles, particularly at night. Symptoms arising from hypermobility may commence at any age (Beighton et al. 1989b); however, Kirk et al. (1967) described a study in which three-quarters of hypermobile subjects had developed symptoms before the age of 15. A feature of normal growth and development is increasing muscle strength (Malina 1985), and in general joint laxity declines with age (Grahame 1999). These normal developmental changes in the soft tissues may be one of the reasons that some hypermobile teenagers experience an improvement in their symptoms as they get older.

Common symptoms among hypermobile adolescents include joint and muscle aches which are often worse at night, excessive clicking of joints, a history of subluxation or dislocation (particularly of the patella or shoulder), non-specific low back pain, joint effusions, repetitive strain injury (RSI), and a feeling of vulnerability as if the joint may lock or 'go out of place'. Symptoms are often worse the day following vigorous or unusual exercise, or after periods of prolonged inactivity such as a long car journey.

Hypermobility syndrome may mimic juvenile chronic arthritis (Bird and Wright 1978), and it has been reported (Gedalia et al. 1985) that 66% (21) of 32 children with episodic arthritis had generalized joint laxity. A diagnosis of hypermobility syndrome may be appropriate in adolescents who have musculoskeletal complaints and joint laxity but no demonstrable evidence of systemic rheumatological disease, providing they fulfil the Brighton Criteria. Hypermobility syndrome is underdiagnosed (Beighton et al. 1989b) and these children are often dismissed as having teenage growing pains or emotional problems.

A review of hypermobile adolescents who attended our clinic over a 2-year period identified some common traits. As small children, those with hypermobility may have a history of walking or crawling late. Indeed, some never crawl – possibly because of poor stability in the elbow and shoulder, and move around by bottom shuffling. Hypermobile children have difficulty in sitting still for any length of time, probably owing to their inability to find a comfortable, stable position, and they have a tendency to fidget. In the classroom this may result in the child being labelled as inattentive or hyperactive. Adolescents have particular difficulty sitting on high stools in science laboratories, as they offer no back support. The problem can be compounded further if the stools do not have a footrest, so that there can be no weight transference of the body through the legs. The inability to place the feet on a footrest or the ground also compromises the stability of the trunk. Hypermobile children may bruise easily, are often clumsy, have poor coordination, and may fall over more frequently than children with 'normal tissues'.

GROWTH

In adolescence the rapid rate of growth can be the trigger for the onset of problems. When treating the adolescent with hypermobility it is essential to have a thorough understanding of normal developmental characteristics to provide a basis for realistic expectations during management.

During early childhood both boys and girls grow at a similar rate in height and weight. The most rapid rate of growth occurs just before birth and it then remains relatively steady until adolescence. Before adolescence the rate of growth is disproportionate throughout the body: the length of the limbs increases more relative to the trunk, and the centre of gravity moves caudally. The peak growth rate (adolescent growth spurt) occurs approximately 2 years after the onset of puberty (Porter 1989). The onset of puberty is approximately 10.5 years in girls and 12.5 years in boys. During this period of rapid growth there is a disproportionate rate of growth of various body parts, resulting in a change of body shape and proportion. The average girl adds between 6 and 11 cm and boys 7–12 cm to their height during this period. Most girls have reached 99% of their adult height by the age of 15, whereas boys reach adult stature between 18 and 21 years.

During the growth spurt, the growth of the bony elements often outstrips that of the soft tissue elements (Thein 1996). It is this stage in development that tissues become overstressed in a cumulative overload, and many adolescents find that their joints are less lax and movements are stiffer. Many experience muscle tightness, and this may be one of the causes of growing pains in children. Typical postural changes at this time include tight thoracolumbar fascia, tight hamstrings, increased lordosis, decreased abdominal strength and a compensatory thoracic kyphosis. Some hypermobile adolescents will not notice any increase in stiffness, but others will notice a reduction in joint laxity in a range that nevertheless remains hypermobile. As changes occur in the muscles and more sarcomeres (the contractile unit of muscle) are laid down, flexibility may improve again.

Weight increases steadily throughout childhood and adolescence. Peak weight velocity follows peak height velocity by 0.25 years in boys and 0.63 years in girls (Tanner 1966). A study of children throughout puberty noted that boys increase in weight by an average of 113%, and girls by an average of 67% (Buckler 1990). This increase in mass (body weight) substantially increases the ground reaction forces to which the joints are subjected, and the more fragile tissues of the hypermobile child become vulnerable if joint stability is further compromised by poor muscle control.

Increases in muscle mass and strength are proportional to weight gain during adolescence (Thein 1996). A boy's muscle mass will double between the ages of 11 and 17 years, and peak height and muscle growth occur simultaneously. A girl's muscle mass doubles between 9 and 15, and the fastest growth is approximately 6 months after peak height velocity. In both sexes increases in muscle strength closely follow increases in muscle mass, which occur approximately 9–12 months after peak height and weight gain (Porter 1989).

Bone maturation is the process whereby the tissue undergoes changes from the embryonic rudiment of bone to the adult form (Roche 1985). Before puberty chronological age correlates well with bone age. However, during adolescence bone age is closely related to adult maturity levels, so that bone age is related to the timing of puberty and growth in height in an individual (Roche 1985). Hence, two adolescents of the same chronological age can have different levels of bone maturation owing to differences in timing of the onset of puberty.

COMMON PROBLEMS IN THE HYPERMOBILE ADOLESCENT

Adolescents may develop symptoms in any joints, but those frequently cited as a problem area are the back, knees, shoulders and elbows. Hypermobile subjects are particularly susceptible to back pain, and the incidence of lumbar disc prolapse, pars interarticularis defects and even spondylolisthesis occurs with increased frequency in hypermobile individuals (Beighton et al. 1989b).

SPINAL PROBLEMS

Pars interarticularis defects

Spondylolysis is a break or discontinuity in the neural arch. Although it is not a congenital defect, there is a strong familial incidence (Turner and Bianco 1971). The incidence of the appearance of this lesion is greatest between 5½ and 6½ years (Wiltse et al. 1976) but symptoms often appear in adolescence, particularly at the time of the growth spurt (Dyrek et al. 1996). The pars defect is considered to be a stress or fatigue fracture caused by repeated hyperflexion, hyperextension and twisting, and consequently it is more prevalent in the adolescent who plays sport. Spondylolysis has been reported with greater frequency in gymnasts, and Jackson et al. (1976) observed that gymnasts with low back pain initially had negative X-rays that then progressed to evident defects in the pars interarticularis. Diagnosis is made from an oblique radiograph. If a stress fracture is suspected and the standard view X-rays appear normal, a bone scan may be required to discount the possibility of a spondylolysis. Spondylolysis has also been reported with greater frequency in a variety of sports, including dancing, tennis, cricket (particularly bowlers), swimming, hurdling and diving.

The stress fracture creates a potential area of instability and symptoms are initially exacerbated by sporting activities, but may become more constant if the defect is not identified. Commonly the teenager will experience pain on flexion or extension that may be reduced if they contract their transversus abdominis muscle before doing active movements. If it is identified in the early stages, conservative treatment of rest followed by controlled activity is successful in the majority of cases. Improving the strength and control of the local muscles that stabilize the lumbar spine and pelvis is an essential part of the management. These lesions can take up to 16 months to heal (Dyrek et al. 1996), but some adolescents may have symptoms severe enough to need surgery.

Spondylolisthesis

A spondylolisthesis occurs when there is a separation of the pars interarticularis defect and a forward slip of one vertebra on another. This condition is more likely to occur in the adolescent growth spurt. The adolescent presents with back pain that may be referred to the legs, loss of lumbar lordosis and hamstring spasm. Diagnosis is made from a lateral radiograph. A slip of 25% or less (grade 1) and even a slip of 50% (grade 2) can often be treated successfully with exercises to improve the muscles that control and stabilize the lumbar spine and pelvis. Larger slips (grades 3 and 4) may require surgery.

Lumbar disc lesions

The increased ligamentous laxity in hypermobility can create greater stresses on the lumbar intervertebral discs, particularly at the end of range of physiological movements. Structures that help to restrain lumbar spine movement include the facet joints, the interspinous ligaments and the discs themselves. The spine does not have the protection from 'normal tight' tissues and the discs are vulnerable to the strains of daily life. Disc damage may be due to a single traumatic incident or result from the repetitive microtrauma and strains to which it is subjected

during everyday activities. Between 30 and 60% of adolescents with disc problems report an association with significant trauma (Grieve 1988a).

A feature of adolescent disc problems is the severity of their objective signs in comparison with adults. They often present with back pain and unilateral leg pain (although it may be bilateral). Movements and activities that increase intradiscal pressure, such as coughing, sneezing, sitting and lifting weights, aggravate the pain. The pain is often reduced in the lying position because the intradiscal pressure is less when axial loading on the spine is reduced. These individuals often have a loss of lumbar lordosis, a lateral shift, and straight-leg raising can be limited to below 30° on the affected side and 45–65° on the unaffected side. In severe cases neurological deficit may develop.

Management of an adolescent disc problem is normally conservative, and surgical intervention should only be considered if there are significant neurological changes. There is tremendous potential for healing and shrinkage of herniated disc material in the adolescent, although healing times can be slow, particularly in the hypermobile. Treatment programmes may include manual mobilization techniques as well as exercises to brace the spine.

Vigorous manipulation of a hypermobile spine that lacks normal tight ligamentous control may put excessive strain on the disc and create further damage, potentially turning a bulging disc into a herniation. Excessive rotational forces are likely to be the most damaging and should be avoided in the hypermobile adolescent.

Non-specific low back pain

Non-specific low back pain is a common problem in hypermobile adolescents and occurs in the absence of demonstrable radiological change or identifiable back pathology. A prospective study of 102 cases of backache (age range 16–70 years) and their relationship to ligamentous laxity was reported by Howes and Isdale (1971). The majority of patients with no definite diagnosis had joint laxity, and Howes and Isdale used the term the 'loose back syndrome'. Other authors have identified similar syndromes (Chabot 1962, Hirsch et al. 1969). Non-specific low back pain often starts in adolescence, when the teenager complains of recurrent low back pain. Neurological signs are absent and examination of the individual reveals they have an increased lumbar lordosis or a sway-back type posture. Relief of symptoms with manipulative treatment is usually only temporary, with longer-lasting improvement gained from isometric back exercises (Howes and Isdale 1971).

Adolescents with hypermobility who suffer with non-specific low back pain often have poor function of the deep trunk and back muscles that help to stabilize the spine, control intersegmental movement and maintain a balanced spine and pelvis. This control is frequently inadequate in static postures and is compromised further during daily functional activities, particularly those that are performed at speed or include a change in the direction of motion. These teenagers need a specific programme aimed at training the muscles of the spine and pelvis to assist in bracing the spine and controlling the forces that affect it.

TRAINING LUMBAR CONTROL IN THE ADOLESCENT HYPERMOBILE

Primary training

The first is a cognitive stage where the individual needs to gain a high level of awareness of finding a lumbar spine neutral position and training the deep muscles. A feature of hypermobility is poor kinaesthesia and reduced proprioception (Hall et al. 1995), so that even finding lumbar spine neutral can be challenging. Hypermobile teenagers often find it particularly difficult to find lumbar spine neutral in four-point kneeling, and may need to start in a supine position to train independence of the pelvis and lower lumbar spine from the thoracic spine and hips without global

muscle substitution. As soon as possible training should be done in sitting or standing, where increased proprioception will be helpful.

Once lumbar spine neutral can be achieved the individual progresses to train lateral costal and diaphragmatic breathing, maintaining lumbar spine neutral.

The next stage is training the middle and lower fibres of transversus abdominis and the pelvic floor. The patient is instructed to draw the lower abdomen 'up and in' without any global muscle substitution. Training with a pressure biofeedback unit in a supine position is often helpful, but as soon as possible the training must be done in weight-bearing and functional postures. When the patient can successfully facilitate transversus abdominis, the next stage is to facilitate bilateral activation of lumbar multifidus, with co-contraction of transversus abdominis while maintaining lumbar spine neutral and controlling lateral costal diaphragmatic breathing (O'Sullivan 2000).

Contractions of the local muscles should be performed as a low load hold, and if global muscle substitution or fatigue occurs the patient must stop the activity. Training requires great concentration and should be performed at least once a day in a quiet environment. The patient begins by holding the contraction for 10 seconds (or less if very weak) and gradually tries to increase the length of low-level hold up to 60 seconds.

Secondary training

This phase of motor training is focused on controlling the particular movements that give the teenager pain, or where they feel vulnerable. Initially training is done in lumbar spine neutral and later progresses to training during normal lumbar spine movement. Adolescents need the exercises to be interesting and challenging, so that the use of equipment such as wobble cushions, gymnastic balls and long D-rolls is often successful. Training must also encompass any sporting or recreational activities in which the teenager participates, and stabilizing exercises are given to maintain intersegmental control at different speeds of motion and sudden changes of direction.

CERVICAL SPINE – ACUTE WRY NECK

An acute torticollis (wry neck) is a common problem in those with hypermobility and often starts in adolescence. It is a painful unilateral condition that often manifests on rising in the morning, particularly in teenagers who sleep prone with their head rotated and extended. A sudden movement of the head can also cause the neck to become 'stuck'. These individuals have poor control of their deep neck stabilizing muscles, so that a sudden overstretching of the neck may cause partial subluxation of the facets, or torn muscles or ligaments (Beighton et al. 1989c).

The condition is characterized by an antalgic posture of flexion and side flexion away from the painful side. Movements towards the side of pain are restricted and painful. There is spasm of sternocleidomastoid and the scaleni muscles, and the articular pillar on the affected side may be very tender to palpation.

An acute wry neck is often self-limiting, so that the pain and muscle spasms ease on their own, usually within a week or two. However, the condition tends to be recurrent, so that episodes of 'locking' occur more frequently, last longer, and become more difficult to help. The pain and restricted movement are debilitating, so that the individual is unable to exercise, play sport, and many normal daily activities are temporarily impossible.

Palpation of the apophyseal joints underlying the muscle spasm will reveal one or two joints that have become hypomobile and acutely tender. The joint stiffness and spasm usually respond well to gentle manual treatment. The use of a vigorous thrust technique is unwise because of the excessive laxity of the unaffected joints (Grieve 1988a). Unless a therapist can confidently localize a manipulative technique to the specific hypomobile segment in an otherwise hypermobile neck, a thrust technique should be avoided as it may cause facet subluxation or overstretch soft tissues.

The most important aspect of managing an acute wry neck is the prevention of recurrences. This is done by specifically training the deep neck flexor muscles that control intersegmental movement in the cervical spine. Training starts with the teenager in supine, their occiput supported on a folded towel so that their neck is in a neutral position. They are taught to do a gentle nod of the head to facilitate the deep neck flexors without substitution from the global stabilizers of sternocleidomastoid and the scaleni. Training is enhanced by the use of a pressure biofeedback unit. The emphasis is on precision and control, the aim being to produce a low-load contraction and hold for 10 seconds, repeated 10 times comfortably (Jull 1997). Once good control in supine has been achieved, they progress to working the deep neck flexors in functional positions such as sitting and standing, and eventually in positions adopted during their daily activities and sporting pastimes.

In addition, it is important to incorporate postural and scapular training. Poor patterns of neuromuscular control in the shoulder girdle muscles can create painful dysfunction in the cervical spine (Jull 2001). Posture should be corrected from the pelvis upwards, and includes attaining an optimal position for the lumbar and thoracic curves with good control of the scapula. Particular attention needs to be paid to the control of the middle and lower fibres of trapezius and serratus anterior. Training of the scapular stabilizers should be low load, performed in a pain-free range and performed short of fatigue.

Many adolescents with hypermobility have difficulty in contracting the scapular stabilizers because of poor proprioception and kinaesthesia. Facilitation of the muscles can often be achieved with the use of EMG biofeedback, visual feedback from a mirror, taping, active assisted exercise and proprioceptive neuromuscular facilitation (PNF) patterning.

HIP

One of the drawbacks of the Beighton scoring system for hypermobility is that it assesses movements at specific joints and ignores other joints that often become symptomatic in hypermobility. The hip and shoulder are both ball and socket joints that normally exhibit a large range of movement and may exhibit excessive range in hypermobile subjects, but do not feature on the Beighton scoring system.

A problem encountered by hypermobile adolescents is a snapping or clicking hip. This can develop secondary to intra- or extra-articular causes. Intra-articular causes include loose bodies, a labral tear, osteocartilaginous exostosis and synovial chondromatosis (Micheli 1983). The commonest extra-articular cause of a clicking hip is the snapping of the iliotibial band over the greater trochanter. Other soft tissue causes are the iliopsoas tendon over the iliopectineal eminence, the iliofemoral ligaments over the femoral head, and the long head of biceps over the ischial tuberosity (Sanders and Nemeth 1996).

Although a clicking hip is a common phenomenon in a hypermobile adolescent the click may or may not be associated with pain (Sanders and Nemeth 1996). In some cases the click is caused by excessive femoral head translation (in an anterior or posterior direction) that is associated with poor control of the muscles of the hip and pelvis. Excessive anterior femoral glide occurs when there is tightness of the posterior capsule and during flexion the femoral head moves anteriorly (Sahrmann 2002). It is often a feature in those with a sway-back posture who stand in postural hip extension. Anterior femoral glide can be observed when the supine patient performs hip flexion or a straight-leg raise. Hip flexion may be restricted or painful at about 90°, and a click may be reproduced when the individual moves the leg actively from a flexed position to neutral. The pain and click can often be reduced by the therapist placing a posteriorly directed force on the femoral head.

The problem is managed by addressing the muscle imbalances of the hip, pelvis and lumbar spine. Those with an anterior femoral glide often have a weak iliopsoas (particularly if they stand in postural hip extension), weak gluteus medius and maximus and tight hamstrings. It can also be associated with overactivity of tensor fascia lata and a tight iliotibial band.

When rehabilitating the hip in a hypermobile adolescent, closed chain exercise is preferable because the weight-bearing component stimulates the mechanoreceptors around the joint, improving muscular contraction. Small range extension in supine with the leg over the side of the bed, the knee flexed to 90° and the foot on the floor is an effective way of facilitating gluteus medius and maximus (Carr and Shepherd 1982). As soon as is viable, the muscles should be exercised as closely as possible to their functional and sporting activities. Retraining the hip muscles must also include an evaluation of timing of muscle contraction and coordination in walking gait and running if the teenager plays sport.

SHOULDER

The shoulder is the most mobile joint in the body, but its greater flexibility is at the expense of stability. Shoulders that are quite lax may be completely stable, whereas those without major laxity can become unstable. Gymnasts may have extreme shoulder flexibility but have sufficient stability to allow them to perform compromising movements such as a unilateral handstand. However, those with generalized hypermobility may be predisposed to shoulder instability.

Glenohumeral instability can range from a vague sense of loss of shoulder function and control to a frank instability due to a traumatic dislocation. Atraumatic instability of the shoulder can become symptomatic in adolescence and is seen more commonly in girls than boys. The individual may have had repeated episodes of recurrent transient subtle subluxations which eventually progress to atraumatic dislocations. Some hypermobile adolescents are able to dislocate or sublux their shoulders voluntarily, and sometimes do this as a 'party trick'. The condition can be unilateral, but is often bilateral in those with excessive ligamentous laxity.

There are a number of reasons why hypermobility can predispose to instability. An extensive joint capsule may allow humeroscapular positions outside the range of balance stability, and poor neuromuscular control may fail to position the scapula to balance the net humeral joint reaction force. An excessively compliant capsule with relatively weak rotator cuff muscles will also reduce the stability of the joint. The instability is most prevalent in mid-range positions and activities of daily living, so that simple actions such as putting on a coat or reaching for a pen can cause the shoulder to sublux.

When examining the hypermobile adolescent with suspected instability it is essential to assess every position where they feel vulnerable or as if the shoulder 'will go out of place'. Jerking, clicking and clunking are noted, and the scapula position observed at the point in range where the instability is dominant. Faulty humeroscapular patterns in combination with poor rotator cuff control are usually the key elements. Neuromuscular control cannot be restored surgically, and these patients require intensive rehabilitation and muscle training to restore normal functional stability.

The patient requires a well constituted, prolonged reconditioning programme that is tailored specifically to their neuromuscular dysfunction. There are two aspects to muscle retraining of the glenohumeral joint. First, the rotator cuff, which compresses the humeral head into the glenoid, must be strengthened, and second, stability is aided by regaining neuromuscular control of humeroscapular positions. Stability must be achieved in all glenohumeral positions, with particular emphasis on those positions where the patient feels vulnerable. It can take several months of conscientiously performing a quality programme for full stability to be achieved. Some

teenagers may need emotional support or counselling to help them understand that surgery is unlikely to be helpful, and that reduction of symptoms will only be possible through their own hard work. They must be encouraged to stop voluntarily subluxing or popping their shoulders out, and try to avoid activities and positions that threaten their shoulder's stability.

Other shoulder conditions, such as impingement, can occur secondarily to instability and this can complicate the clinical picture.

Facilitation of the scapular stabilizers and rotator cuff may be enhanced with the use of EMG biofeedback, PNF patterning and the use of mirrors and taping. Exercises in weight-bearing will also help to improve proprioception.

KNEE

Knee pain is a common manifestation in adolescents, particularly those with hypermobility. Twenty-five per cent of the population suffers from patellofemoral pain at some time in their lives (McConnell and Fulkerson 1996), and it is particularly common in the athletic population and in those with hypermobility.

Anterior knee pain

The causes of patellofemoral pain are multifactorial and can be either structural or non-structural. Structural factors include femoral anteversion, increased Q angle, patella alta, patella baja, genu valgum, genu varum, excessive foot pronation and genu recurvatum (Malek and Mangine 1981), which can affect the balance of the soft tissues surrounding the patella. The latter two are common clinical features of hypermobility which will make the individual more susceptible to anterior knee pain.

An alteration in the balance of soft tissue structures that surround the patella is a major contributory factor, as movement of the patella is controlled by this and the shape of the articular surfaces and the supporting muscles. Malalignment of the patella due to biomechanical faults affects the tracking of the patella during knee movements. This alters forces through the joint, which can cause damage to the articular cartilage. The articular cartilage is avascular and aneural, so that when degeneration occurs in the deep and middle layers of the cartilage there are changes in the energy absorption capacity of that cartilage. This results in transference of weight from the articular cartilage to the richly innervated subchondral bone, and hence an increase in intraosseous pressure. Degenerative changes in the superficial layer of cartilage can irritate the synovium, causing synovitis and pain (Fulkerson and Hungerford 1990).

During the growth spurt, the muscles and soft tissues can become relatively tight and a decrease in flexibility of the lateral retinaculum, hamstrings, rectus femoris, gastrocnemius, soleus and tensor fascia lata (TFL) can adversely affect the tracking of the patella and become a trigger for the onset of symptoms. At the start of knee flexion, if the lateral retinaculum is short it comes under stress and the patella is drawn into the trochlea. The tension increases further as the iliotibial band (ITB) moves posterior to the epicondyle of the femur. As knee flexion increases the ITB pulls posteriorly on the already shortened retinaculum. These changes in the soft tissues cause lateral tracking and a lateral tilt of the patella (Fulkerson and Hungerford 1990). Vastus medialis oblique (VMO) is a dynamic medial stabilizer of the patella, and if it weakens it is unable to resist the pull of any tight lateral structures.

Episodic joint effusions can be a feature of hypermobility syndrome. VMO is inhibited by joint effusion (Spencer et al. 1984) and, when present, individuals rapidly develop weakness of VMO, which becomes only phasically active, so that abnormal patellar tracking occurs. Pelvic muscle imbalances and abnormal gait patterns can also lead to patellofemoral problems. Examination of anterior knee pain in hypermobility requires an in-depth assessment of the length, strength and control of the muscles and soft tissues that surround the patella, so that appropriate rehabilitation programmes can be implemented that address the relevant imbalances.

Patellofemoral instability

Patellofemoral instability is a variant of patellofemoral pain syndromes. It is more common in females, those with generalized hypermobility, and those who have patella alta, a Q angle greater than 20°, dysplasia of the trochlea and patella, and hyperextension of the knee (Insall 1979, Hughston 1989). The patella may sublux laterally or dislocate, and the patient exhibits apprehension when the patella is passively moved laterally. Patellar instability can be devastating to the articular cartilage, although Stanitski (1995) found that hypermobile individuals were 2.5 times less likely to suffer articular surface damage with patellar dislocation.

Physiotherapy intervention aimed at trying to optimize biomechanical alignment and addressing the soft tissue imbalances of the patella is often successful. Treatment includes a strengthening programme for VMO and exercises to improve pelvic stability. Those with hypermobility also need to emphasize exercises aimed at improving proprioception and kinaesthesia.

Genu recurvatum

Excessive hyperextension of the knee can result in nipping or trapping of the infrapatellar fat pad in the knee. The patient presents with tenderness and puffiness around the inferior pole of the patella. The pain is worse on standing, particularly if the individual hyperextends the knee, and is reproduced by extension overpressure. Malalignment of the patella can cause the inferior pole to be displaced posteriorly, so that the fat pad is compressed. Retraining the quadriceps, hamstrings and stability muscles of the pelvis is a key feature in the management of this problem and is best performed in weight-bearing positions to ensure improvement in the control of knee hyper-extension in a functional position. Strenuous work of the quadriceps alone could simply reinforce the hyperextension of the knee and exacerbate the problem.

FOOT

Abnormal pronation of the foot is defined as an abnormal pronation of the entire foot which occurs at the subtalar joint (Wilson 1906), and it is responsible for more chronic low-grade symptomatology in the lower leg than any other type of foot problem (Root et al. 1977). During locomotion the foot may function around an abnormally pronated position, or may move in the direction of pronation at the time when it should be supinating. There are a number of common congenital and developmental foot deformities which are compensated for by abnormal pronation. The commoner deformities include forefoot varus, rearfoot varus and ankle joint equinus. There are also a number of structural deformities extrinsic to the foot compensated for by abnormal pronation, and these include tibia vara, internal tibial torsion, internal femoral torsion, congenitally shortened gastroc-soleus and hamstrings. In addition to any congenital or developmental deformities individuals with generalized hypermobility have a greater tendency to overpronation owing to the laxity of their ligaments, poor control of the phasic muscles which stabilize during gait, and the 'creep' effect that makes soft tissues elongate under load in a weight-bearing position (Root et al. 1977).

Excessive pronation increases forces across the foot and can lead to symptomatology and even subluxation of some of the joints. A stable foot is essential, and instability created by overpronation readily affects other joints. As the subtalar joint pronates it causes internal rotation of the tibia and femur, thereby creating abnormal function in the lower limb and pelvis. Normal foot function in an individual with generalized hypermobility will be compromised if they have an unstable foot, and this will have a detrimental effect on their ability to stabilize other joints of the lower limb and pelvis.

When the bones of the foot become unstable, the forces across the bones create movement of the joints in the direction of the application of those forces acting upon them. If these forces produce joint movement they increase hypermobility. The abnormal shifting of the weight-bearing bones of the foot causes excessive shearing between the bones and the surrounding soft tissues, and adaptive changes occur in both the bones and the soft tissues. In the hypermobile adolescent the bone adapts rapidly by changing shape, and new bone is laid down in accordance with requirements of function and in accordance with the transmission of forces through the bone. As growth occurs rapidly during adolescence, permanent osseous deformity can occur.

During the gait cycle, when the foot first hits the ground it needs to become a mobile adaptor to make full ground contact, and this is normally the time when the foot pronates. Further propulsion requires the foot to become a rigid lever, and the tarsal bones must become locked together by the osseous locking mechanisms which occur as the foot is supinated. This action stabilizes the major functional joints of the foot. The stability of the foot is reinforced by the contraction of the stance phase muscles (Root et al. 1977). The integrity of the joints is maintained and the shear forces are reduced to prevent symptomatology.

If the foot remains abnormally pronated during propulsion the normal osseous locking mechanisms within the tarsus are less efficient. The tarsus becomes unstable and the phasic muscles are unable to sufficiently stabilize. As the heel lifts the forces supported by the forefoot cause the individual bones to move abnormally relative to each other and joint stability is diminished. The abnormal forces may eventually cause the joints to sublux.

Hypermobility of the foot has been linked to many different clinical foot disorders, and common problems include hyperkeratoses on the toes and plantar surfaces of the feet, metatarsalgia, plantar fasciitis, hallux abductovarus, hallux limitus, hallux rigidus, muscle fatigue, and strains in the lower leg (Root et al. 1977). Many of these problems start to become symptomatic during adolescence owing to the rapid growth phase and the greater body weight, which increases the forces sustained by the feet.

Some hypermobile adolescents may be helped by an exercise programme aimed at improving the function of the muscles of the lower limb, but others require some form of orthosis that will help to control the hypermobility and improve the stability of the foot. The prescription of an orthotic for an adolescent with hypermobility must take into account any congenital or developmental deformity, as well as the poor proprioception and skin fragility that are a feature of hypermobility. If an orthosis made of a soft, flexible material is supplied, it can make joint proprioception and kinaesthesia more difficult for the hypermobile adolescent, and this can be improved by the use of a firmer material or rigid device. However, some hypermobile individuals are unable to tolerate a rigid device because of the fragility of their tissues, and require appropriate materials to counteract this.

Abnormal pronation is greater in running owing to the increase in ground reaction forces and an increase in functional limb varus. A hypermobile adolescent may therefore be symptom free when walking, but complain of pain and muscle strains when running. The use of well fitting, supportive footwear that is appropriate to the particular sport is essential, especially during the rapid growth phase.

PSYCHOSOCIAL FACTORS

The physical changes that occur during adolescence are accompanied by emotional and psychological development, which can make it a confusing and difficult time for a teenager. An adolescent with hypermobility will not necessarily experience symptoms, but the onset of unexplained pain may be frightening and can cause additional emotional distress. It is helpful for adolescents to understand the nature of their problem and to learn that it can be managed successfully. The development of fear/avoidance behaviour in those who have hypermobility syndrome needs to be identified and addressed. If a movement or activity becomes painful an individual may avoid performing various actions because they fear they are doing irreversible damage to their body. As movement patterns alter, elements within the musculoskeletal system adapt so that there is greater dysfunction and pain is provoked more easily. In turn, the individual restricts his activities further and a cycle develops which becomes increasingly difficult to change. An understanding of the physiological condition and reassurance that it is important to maintain as normal a lifestyle as possible is essential in the prevention of chronic pain.

Compliance

Successful management of the hypermobile adolescent is dependent on the compliance of the individual.

Compliance can be difficult and challenging to achieve in a teenager. At our clinic we have found the following points helpful:

1. Listen carefully to the patient and ensure that you fully understand the extent and nature of his or her problems. It is essential to realize the impact of their problems on school, social and home life. The teenager will have greater confidence in you if they think you understand their problem.
2. Talk directly to the patient and keep eye contact. Teenagers under 16 years of age should be accompanied by a parent or guardian, but do not ignore the adolescent and talk solely to the adult. It is important to build a good basis for communication with the teenager from the start. If the parent answers questions for the

adolescent, gently tell them that you would like the child to answer, and that they will be given an opportunity to comment or ask questions during the examination.

3. Explain the problem clearly to both the patient and their parent. Teenagers are intelligent and have a natural curiosity. They are more likely to follow an exercise regimen and other lifestyle changes if they understand the need for and the likely benefits of a management programme.

4. A positive attitude from the physiotherapist is essential. The adolescent must understand that they can take back control of their problem themselves if they are prepared to put the work in first. Emphasize that many hypermobile adolescents keep symptoms at bay and partake in the same activities as their peers once they have trained the appropriate muscle groups and improved their exercise tolerance.

5. Set realistic goals for exercise programmes, general fitness and lifestyle adjustments. Give encouragement and praise achievement.

6. Exercises given as homework must be pain free. If an exercise hurts, the teenager is unlikely to continue with it and quickly loses confidence in the rehabilitation strategy. It is usually possible to find an exercise that is not painful to perform. We rarely give a patient more than three exercises at one time and expect that they will have achieved a pre-agreed target by their next attendance. Once a patient can do an exercise well it is modified or replaced with one that is more challenging.

7. Make the exercise fun and interactive. We have found the use of EMG and pressure biofeedback, jelly cushions, wobble boards, gymnastic balls and other equipment effective and popular with teenagers.

8. Remember that exercises take time to work. Explain this to the patient and set a realistic timescale for when you would expect to see some improvement in symptoms. During this time it is quite normal to have some days that are not as good as others, and encourage the adolescent to continue with the programme on both good and bad days.

9. When dealing with the anxious parents of a hypermobile teenager encourage them not to become overprotective, and stress that it is important and healthy for their child to do as many normal activities as possible. If a particular activity presents a recurring problem, discuss ways of modifying it so that the adolescent can continue. As the overall condition of the teenager improves with treatment and exercise, many activities that were once difficult or inhibited by pain become pain free.

SPORT

Adolescents with hypermobility should be encouraged to take regular exercise and play sport. The benefits of sport for the hypermobile include improving cardiovascular fitness, improvements in muscle strength and control, coordination and proprioception, and a feeling of wellbeing. There is no one particular form of exercise that has been proved to be superior to any other for those with hypermobility, but it is important that it is an activity or form of exercise that the teenager enjoys and feels comfortable doing. Although swimming is excellent exercise for the hypermobile, it is advisable to also include some form of regular exercise that is weight-bearing to increase bone loading and improve proprioception. There are many benefits of playing team sports and taking part in exercise with other adolescents, but playing contact sports such as rugby may be inadvisable for some individuals with hypermobility syndrome. Those with hypermobility will need a training programme that includes muscle control work specific to their individual needs and the physical demands of their particular sport. If sport or exercise is painful, the adolescent should be carefully assessed to identify any specific training needs.

Liaising with the individual's PE teachers, sports coaches or trainers can be useful. It is important that those involved with teaching or coaching an adolescent who has hypermobility are aware of the condition and watch out for potential problems. It is helpful if hypermobile adolescents are able to take part in sport at school with their friends and peers.

LIFESTYLE ADAPTATIONS

Adaptations and changes in lifestyle and habits can make everyday activities more comfortable.

The use of a good backpack to carry schoolwork and other items will reduce the stresses on the spine and upper limbs. Study positions at home and school are frequently triggers for the onset of pain. Advice on sitting positions for schoolwork and studying are essential. The provision of items such as a supportive adjustable chair, writing slopes, copyholders, pens with a thick grip and ergonomic keyboards may be helpful. However, even when a work or study position is optimal, prolonged sitting can cause discomfort, and over a period of time soft tissue adaptations

---

Case study

A 15-year-old student presented with a 2-year history of problems. She gave a history of pain in the interscapular area which spread to the neck and low back. A year after the onset of her problem she was also getting pain in both hips and knees. She had a series of investigations, including X-rays, blood tests, MRI and CT scans, which were all normal. Three months after the onset of symptoms she was advised to stop all sport and any activities that exacerbated her condition. The adolescent had received treatment (exercise, manipulation, traction, medication and electrotherapy) from a variety of practitioners with no success, and her problem had become so severe that in the previous 3 months she had only felt well enough to attend school on 12 occasions. She was referred to physiotherapy by a consultant, but was reluctant to come for treatment as previous treatments had been unsuccessful and had even worsened her symptoms.

On examination she had poor posture, with obvious lack of control of the spinal and pelvic stabilizers. She stood with both knees in hyperextension and with bilateral pronated feet. The head was in a forward position, she had an increased thoracic kyphosis, and poor control of the scapular stabilizers. Her spinal movements were generally good and she was able to bend forward and place both hands flat on the floor. However, she had difficulty in returning to the upright position and had to place her hands on her thighs to assist her return to upright standing. She demonstrated excessive flexibility in other joints and scored 7/9 on the Beighton scale.

The range of neck movements was also good, but she had particular difficulty in returning the extended neck to a neutral position and had to use a hand to support her neck. Neurological examination was normal. She was hypersensitive and jumpy on palpation of the spine.

Management
She was given a careful explanation of JHS and, in discussion with the girl and her parents, a management strategy was developed. She was anxious about trying any form of exercise as this had always aggravated her symptoms in the past. We explained that the exercises should be pain free while she was performing them. We also told her that she would start to notice a difference in her symptoms after about a month, but it would take

approximately 8 months of training to regain full muscle control. On the first attendance she was taught low-load abdominal bracing with the help of a pressure biofeedback. On her second attendance there was no improvement in her symptoms but she could do specific deep abdominal bracing and repeat it several times without pain. She was praised for her achievement, and rewarded with a more challenging exercise for the deep abdominal muscles. She was also taught to contract the deep neck flexors and loaned a pressure biofeedback with the aim of improving the deep neck flexor control over the next week. During the following weeks she worked hard to improve trunk stability, and treatment was exercise and advice based. After 5 weeks she reported that she had less pain and could study for longer periods without having to lie down. At the end of 8 weeks she had managed to go to school for 3 weeks without taking a day off. At this point specific soft tissue mobilizations were used to treat trigger points in the upper fibres of trapezius, and she was taught scapular stabilizing exercises.

The trunk stability exercises were progressed to become more challenging and she was loaned various pieces of equipment to make the work interesting and fun. She gradually gained more confidence and began activities aimed at improving her cardiovascular fitness. Initially she started with a brisk 10-minute daily walk and quickly progressed to swimming on a regular basis. Five months after the onset of treatment she reported that she had had no pain in the previous 2 weeks and had returned to most of her normal activities.

Comment
After discussion with the patient's parents, it was noted that the onset of symptoms correlated with a growth spurt. Early on, the patient had been advised to stop all physical activity and consequently had developed considerable muscle weakness, particularly of the stabilizing muscles of the spine and pelvis. The spread of symptoms and lack of improvement with various treatments had caused great anxiety to the girl and her family. The teenager had been dismissed by some as having 'growing pains', or told that it was 'all in the mind'. This is a scenario that we see all too often at our clinic.

can occur. Therefore, advice on regular breaks and gentle stretching exercises to maintain range of movement is useful. Even though a hypermobile teenager has an excessive range of movement, it is important that they maintain their normal range of movement and have good control of movement throughout their hypermobile range.

CONCLUSION

An adolescent with hypermobility syndrome may present with a number of different physical problems. Management must take into account the various physical, emotional and psychological changes that are taking place during the teenage years.

REFERENCES

Apple, D.F. (1985) Adolescent runners. *Clinics in Sports Medicine*, **4**, 641–55.

Beighton, P., Grahame, G. and Bird, H. (1989a) *Hypermobility of Joints*, 2nd edn, p 130. Springer-Verlag.

Beighton, P., Grahame, G. and Bird, H. (1989b) *Hypermobility of Joints*, 2nd edn, p 2–3. Springer-Verlag.

Beighton, P., Grahame, G. and Bird, H. (1989c) *Hypermobility of Joints*, 2nd edn, p 89. Springer-Verlag.

Bird, H.A. and Wright, V. (1978) Joint hypermobility mimicking periarticular juvenile chronic arthritis. *British Medical Journal*, **3**, 402–3.

Buckler, J. (1990) *A Longitudinal Study of Adolescent Growth*. New York: Springer Verlag.

Carr, J. and Shepherd, R. (1982) *A Motor Relearning Program for Stroke*, p. 107. London: Heinemann.

Chabot, J. (1962) *Les Consultations Journalières en Rhumatologie*, p 65. Paris: Masson.

Dyrek, D.A., Micheli, L.J. and Magee, D.J. (1996) Injuries to the thoracolumbar spine and pelvis. In: *Athletic Injuries and Rehabilitation* (J.E. Zachazewski, D. Magee and W.S. Quillen, eds), p. 474. Saunders.

Fulkerson, J. and Hungerford, D. (1990) *Disorders of the Patellofemoral Joint*, 2nd edn. Baltimore: Williams & Wilkins.

Gedalia, A., Person, A.D., Brewer. E.J. and Giannini, E.H. (1985) Juvenile episodic arthralgia and hypermobility. *Journal of Pediatrics*, **107**, 873–6.

Grahame, R. (1999) Joint hypermobility and genetic collagen disorders: are they related? *Archives of Disease in Childhood*, **80**, 188–91.

Grahame, R. and Jenkins, J.M. (1972) Joint hypermobility – asset or liability. *Annals of the Rheumatic Diseases*, **31**, 109–11.

Grieve, G.P. (1988a) *Common Vertebral Joint Problems*, 2nd edn, p. 411. Churchill Livingstone.

Grieve, G.P. (1988b) *Common Vertebral Joint Problems*, 2nd edn, p. 648. Churchill Livingstone.

Hall, M.G., Ferrell, W.R., Sturrock, R.D. et al. (1995) The effect of the hypermobility syndrome on knee joint proprioception. *British Journal of Rheumatology*, **34**, 121–5.

Hirsch, C.J., Jonsson, B. and Lewin, T. (1969) Low back pain in a Swedish female population. *Acta Orthopedica Scandinavica*, **3**, 171–6.

Howes, R.G. and Isdale, I.C. (1971) The loose back: an unrecognized syndrome. *Rheumatology and Physical Medicine*, **11**, 72–7.

Hughston, J. (1989) Patellar subluxation: a recent history. *Clinics in Sports Medicine*, **8**, 153–62.

Insall, J. (1979) Chondromalacia patellae: patella malalignment syndrome. *Orthopedic Clinics of North America*. Orthopedic Clinics of North America.

Jackson, D.W., White, L.L. and Circincione, R.J. (1976) Spondylolysis in the female gymnast. *Clinical Orthopedics*, **117**, 68–73.

Jull, G. (1997) The management of cervicogenic headache. *Manual Therapy*, **2**, 182–90.

Jull, G. (2001) The physiotherapy management of whiplash associated disorders. Proceedings of 2nd IPPA Conference, England.

Kirk, J.A., Ansell, B.M. and Bywaters, E.G.L. (1967) The hypermobility syndrome. Musculoskeletal complaints associated with generalized hypermobility. *Annals of the Rheumatic Diseases*, **26**, 419–25.

Klemp, P., Stevens, J.E. and Isaacs, S. (1984) A hypermobility study in ballet dancers. *Journal of Rheumatology*, **11**, 692–6.

Larsson, L.-G., Baum, J., Muldolkar, G.S. and Kollia, G.D. (1993) Benefits and disadvantages of joint hypermobility among musicians. *New England Journal of Medicine*, **329**, 1079–82.

Malina, R.M. (1985) Growth of muscle tissue and muscle mass. In: *Human Growth: A Comprehensive Treatise* (F. Falkner and J.M. Tanner, eds) 2nd edn, Vol 2. New York: Plenum.

Malek, M. and Mangine, R. (1981) Patellofemoral pain syndromes: a comprehensive and conservative approach. *Journal of Orthopedics and Sports Physical Therapy*, **2**, 108–16.

McConnell, J. and Fulkerson, J. (1996) The knee: patellofemoral and soft tissue injuries. In: *Athletic Injuries and Rehabilitation* (J.E. Zachazewski, D. Magee and W.S. Quillen, eds), p. 701. Saunders.

Micheli, L.J. (1983) Overuse injuries in children's sports: the growth factor. *Orthopedic Clinics of North America*, **14**, 337–61.

O'Sullivan, P.B. (2000) Lumbar segmental 'instability': clinical presentation and specific stabilizing exercise management. *Manual Therapy*, **5**, 2–12.

Porter, R.E. (1989) Normal development of movement and function: child and adolescent. In: *Physical Therapy* (R.M. Scully and M.R. Barnes, eds). Philadelphia: J.B. Lippincott.

Roche, A.F. (1985) Bone growth and maturation. In: *Human Growth: A Comprehensive Treatise* (F. Falkner and J.M. Tanner, eds), 2nd edn, Vol 2. New York: Plenum.

Root, M.L., Orien, W.P. and Weed, J.H. (1977) Normal and abnormal function of the foot. *Clinical Biomechanics*, **II**, 110–25.

Sahrmann, S. (2002) Diagnosis and Treatment of Movement Impairment Syndromes. p. 146. Mosby.

Sanders, B. and Nemeth, W.C. (1996) Hip and thigh injuries. In: *Athletic Injuries and Rehabilitation* (J.E. Zachazewski, D. Magee and W.S. Quillen, eds), pp. 599–622. Saunders.

Spencer, J., Hayes, K. and Alexander, I. (1984) Knee joint effusion and quadriceps reflex inhibition in man. *Archives of Physical Medicine*, **65**, 171–7.

Stanitski, C.L. (1995) Articular hypermobility and chondral injury in patients with acute patellar dislocation. *American Journal of Sports Medicine*, **23**, 146–50.

Tanner, J.M. (1966) Standards from birth to maturity for height, weight, height velocity, and weight velocity: British children. *Archives of Disease in Childhood*, **41**, 454.

Thein, L. (1996) The child and adolescent athlete. In: *Athletic Injuries and Rehabilitation* (J.E. Zachazewski, D. Magee and W.S. Quillen, eds), p 933. Saunders.

Turner, R.H. and Bianco, A.J. (1971) Spondylolysis and spondylolisthesis in children and teenagers. *Journal of Bone and Joint Surgery [American]*, **53A**, 1298.

Wilson, H.A. (1906) Hallux valgus. *American Journal of Orthopedic Surgery*, **3**, 214–30.

Wiltse, L.L., Newman, P.H. and Macnab, I. (1976) Classification of spondylolysis and spondylolisthesis. *Clinical Orthopedics and Related Research*, **117**, 23.

Zaricznyj, B., Shattuck, L.J., Masts, T.S. et al. (1980) Sports-related injuries in school-age children. *American Journal of Sports Medicine*, **8**, 318–23.

6

Physiotherapy assessment of the hypermobile adult

Rosemary Keer

Aims

1. To discuss how joint hypermobility syndrome (JHS) presents in the adult
2. To provide guidelines to aid recognition of the syndrome
3. To discuss possible mechanisms for the production of symptoms reported by JHS patients
4. To discuss possible implications of JHS in the pregnant woman

INTRODUCTION

Joint hypermobility syndrome (JHS), a collection of musculoskeletal symptoms associated with generalized hypermobility of the joints, is under-diagnosed (Beighton et al. 1999) and frequently unrecognized by doctors and physical therapists. Physiotherapists are experienced in performing comprehensive neuromusculoskeletal examinations and, as such, are well placed to identify and treat joint hypermobility syndrome sufferers effectively. However, although physiotherapists are familiar with the joint laxity caused by damage to ligaments in an isolated joint, such as an anterior cruciate-deficient knee, they have less experience of dealing with the consequences of generalized laxity, as seen in the JHS patient. This chapter aims to raise awareness of the condition, to aid recognition and understanding, and to explore possible reasons why generalized hypermobility may cause problems.

RECOGNITION

Recognition and understanding are the most important factors in managing JHS for patient and physiotherapist alike. Recognition is often difficult. One of the main reasons for this would appear to be that JHS patients do not exhibit many of the signs normally associated with painful musculoskeletal conditions. They frequently present with no reduction in range of movement and often have no signs of inflammation (Russek 1999). A large part of the physiotherapist's examination is concerned with the assessment of restricted movement, and when faced with a patient who has a good range of movement there is a danger that it can lead to their condition being misunderstood, as the symptoms do not appear to fit with the signs. At its worst, it can result in the patient being labelled as suffering from a psychological disorder, with unhelpful comments such as 'it is all in the mind' being reported by patients in the clinic and also in the literature (Child 1986, Lewkonia and Ansell 1983).

Physiotherapists, partly because of time constraints, can also be guilty of focusing on the main problem area during the examination, rather than the whole patient, and consequently miss the fact that the patient is displaying generalized hypermobility. Joint hypermobility is common (Larsson et al. 1995) and it is worth remembering that to many, hypermobility poses no problems and can actually be of benefit (Larsson et al. 1993). However, there is a huge spectrum of presentations, ranging from the accomplished ballet dancer and gymnast who demonstrates marked hypermobility without suffering from the syndrome, to someone who is suffering from the syndrome with severe symptoms and may be relatively disabled and reliant on aids or in a wheelchair.

Recognizing JHS can be difficult because patients are often unable to give a reason for the onset of symptoms. Trivial everyday activities can cause significant pain, making them feel that there is something seriously wrong. Recognizing and understanding the condition ensure that the patient is reassured that they are not suffering from a life-threatening disorder, and also that the condition can be successfully managed.

Patients often consult a physiotherapist without a diagnosis of JHS and it is important for a variety of reasons that, when present, the condition is recognized. Patients have often seen many different practitioners, including doctors, physiotherapists, osteopaths, chiropractors and alternative therapists, without having been given a diagnosis, gaining no significant benefit, and in some cases they are actually made worse. This search for help often leaves patients angry with the medical profession, anxious and depressed.

Recognizing the syndrome also ensures that patients can get appropriate treatment.

Cherpel and Marks (1999) state that although joint hypermobility is a common phenomenon, it is possibly undertreated or inappropriately treated owing to a lack of basic knowledge about the condition. At its worst, this can lead to the patient undergoing a battery of unnecessary tests, invasive orthopaedic procedures or inappropriate use of potent antirheumatic drugs (Lewkonia and Ansell 1983), which only serves to increase suffering with no discernible benefit.

There is evidence to suggest that JHS predisposes to several articular and non-articular lesions (El-Shahaly and El-Sherif 1991), and even the early onset of osteoarthritis (OA) (Kirk et al. 1967, Bird et al. 1978). It is important that patients are aware of this possibility and given helpful information and education to help prevent or reduce this potential complication. It is also possible that by recognizing the condition early and implementing appropriate treatment and advice, the JHS patient can be prevented from becoming a chronic pain sufferer.

Many sufferers report that physical therapy in the past has made them worse, and this is almost certainly because the condition was not identified. In JHS the collagenous tissues in the body are less resilient and therefore more vulnerable to injury (Acasuso-Diaz et al. 1993) and musculoskeletal disorders (Bridges et al. 1992). An appreciation of this is necessary to avoid exacerbating symptoms or, even worse, causing further damage. For the physiotherapist it is therefore important to take extra care when handling the hypermobile patient's tissues, both in examination and in treatment. Clinical experience also suggests that the JHS patient takes longer to treat. This is due to the widespread nature of symptoms, the length of time they have had problems – in some cases for many years, which causes them to become deconditioned – and because their tissues take longer to heal (Russek 2000).

HYPERMOBILITY, INSTABILITY AND THE HYPERMOBILITY SYNDROME

Hypermobility is said to be present when there is an increase in the range of movement at a joint beyond the accepted norm. This may apply to one joint in isolation, such as a ligament injury in the knee following trauma. Generalized hypermobility is said to be present when many joints in the body have an increased range of movement. This can be seen in certain groups of people, such as gymnasts and ballet dancers (Gannon and Bird 1999). In this group of people the increased mobility is considered to be the upper extreme of a wide normal variation in joint mobility, some of which may have been gained through training. This can be considered an asset (Larsson et al. 1993), and appears to convey an elegance and grace to their movements. Many individuals with generalized hypermobility do not appear to have any problems associated with their increased flexibility.

Joint hypermobility syndrome, however, is defined as generalized joint laxity with associated musculoskeletal complaints in the absence of any systemic disease (Kirk et al. 1967). JHS has been shown to be an inherited form of generalized connective tissue disorder (Grahame 1999). It is presumed that it is the increased mobility that is contributing to the complaints of musculoskeletal symptoms. However, Kirk et al. (1967) found that a higher hypermobility joint score did not always

accompany severe complaints or a more widespread pattern of referral. It is not known what causes the pain associated with JHS, but several theories have been proposed. Some believe pain is produced as a result of joint microtrauma from overuse and misuse (Kirk et al. 1967, Russek 2000) of tissues that have an inherent weakness in their collagen structure. Child (1986) suggests pain is due to sensory nerve endings which are overstimulated by stretch, but which are poorly supported by collagen fibrils and hence are overstimulated as the lax capsule is stretched. It is clear that the pain associated with hypermobility may begin as a localized joint pain, but frequently develops into a chronic pain with alterations in central nervous system processing. There is also evidence to suggest that dysfunction in the autonomic nervous system may play a part (Gazit et al. 2003).

From a physiotherapy management point of view, it is helpful to look in more detail at the theories behind hypermobility or increased joint mobility and why it can sometimes cause problems. One of the mechanisms involved in the development of symptoms is likely to be a lack of control of the hypermobile joint range. This will make it more susceptible to injury from overuse and misuse, or even normal use. The issue then is one of joint stability. Stability is dynamic and defined as the ability to transfer load effectively, and it follows that a stable joint is less likely to cause problems.

Panjabi (1992a) proposes a model of spinal stability and movement which can be applied to other joints in the body. He suggests that joint stability is dependent on three subsystems which are functionally interdependent (Fig. 6.1):

1. Passive musculoskeletal subsystem, which includes the bones and the shape of the articulating surfaces, ligaments, joint capsules and the passive mechanical properties of muscle;
2. Active musculoskeletal subsystem, which consists of the muscles and tendons surrounding the joint;

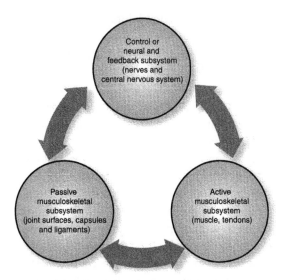

Figure 6.1 Components contributing to joint stability (after Panjabi 1992)

(a)

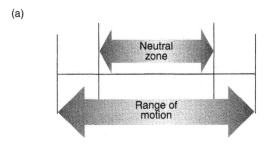

(b)

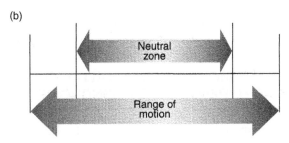

Figure 6.2 (a) The neutral zone (after Panjabi 1992); (b) The neutral zone increased

3. Control or neural and feedback subsystem, which consists of the various force and motion transducers located in ligaments, tendons and muscles and the neural control centres.

In addition, Panjabi (1992b) (Fig. 6.2) describes a neutral zone, which is that part of the physiological motion, measured from the neutral position, within which motion is produced with a minimal internal resistance. It is the zone of high flexibility or laxity. This neutral zone can be increased by injury, degeneration and weakness of stability muscles (Fig. 6.2).

From our knowledge of the effects of deficient collagen synthesis it is possible to hypothesize how joint stability may be compromised in JHS. Less restraint and control may be provided by increased extensibility of ligaments, capsules and muscles, leading to a deficiency in the passive system and an increase in the neutral zone. Decreased muscle tone and tensile strength in the tendons will affect the active subsystem, and deficient proprioception may lead to problems in the neural and feedback subsystem, leading to abnormal motor control.

Panjabi (1992a) defined clinical spinal instability as a significant decrease in the capacity of the stabilizing system of the spine to maintain intervertebral neutral zones within physiological limits, so that there is no neurological dysfunction, major deformity or incapacitating pain.

Panjabi (1992b) found from an in vitro study and mathematical model that simulated muscle force was effective in reducing the neutral zone, and hypothesized that muscles are capable of restoring stability after injury. It has been proposed that there are two muscle systems involved in the maintenance of spinal stability (Bergmark 1989). These are the 'global muscle system', made up of large superficial muscles which produce spinal movement without attaching directly to the spine, and the 'local muscle system', i.e. smaller deeper muscles which attach to the lumbar vertebrae and provide segmental stability and control rather than movement (O'Sullivan 2000). Spinal stability is achieved through coordinated muscle recruitment of both systems.

This concept of spinal stability currently provides the basis for physiotherapy management of JHS, which is concerned with improving the stability and control of hypermobile joints. There has been little research to validate this approach, although the studies by Barton and Bird (1996) and Kerr et al. (2000) have shown positive effects from a joint stabilization programme in JHS patients. In addition, work by Richardson et al. (1999) and O'Sullivan (2000) on segmental stabilization is providing evidence of the efficacy of this approach in the treatment of low back pain, and much of this can be applied to the management of JHS.

This hypothesis of instability may go some way to explain why the JHS patient suffers pain from seemingly normal or everyday activities, and why they appear to prefer resting at the end of range where they feel more secure. It may also explain why the hypermobility syndrome affects many more females than males. Females have a tendency to increased range of movement and less muscle bulk, although a hormonal or genetic factor may also be involved. This hypothesis does not, however, explain why some hypermobile individuals have no problems whereas others have many, and further research in this area is clearly needed.

ASSESSMENT OF THE JHS PATIENT

Recognizing JHS as a cause for a patient's symptoms can be difficult. A range of characteristics which can help the physiotherapist identify and diagnose JHS are discussed. These have been identified from clinical experience and research. It should be stressed that patients will not suffer all the symptoms discussed.

The gender of the patient can be relevant, as JHS is more common in females than males. Grahame (1986) found that 2% of 9275 patients attending a rheumatology clinic were diagnosed with JHS, and of these 85% were female.

Ethnicity is also important, as different races have different mobility characteristics. Joint hypermobility varies in prevalence from 5% of a cohort of blood donors in the USA (Jessee et al. 1980) to between 25% and 38% in a cohort of students in Iraq (Al-Rawi et al. 1985). Asian Indians were found by Wordsworth et al. (1987) to be significantly more mobile than English Caucasians.

The dominant side is usually less mobile than the non-dominant side (Verhoeven et al. 1999), owing to the tendency for more muscle development on the dominant side through increased use, or possibly better motor control.

Symptoms

If the patient has arrived without a diagnosis of JHS, recognition is often difficult because the patient looks well and moves well. It is tempting to think they are overemphasizing their pain and complaints. This is often because they have been badly managed in the past by medical practitioners and other health professionals who have failed to listen to them and heed their message. They need to feel that they have finally found someone who will listen to them and believe them. It is advisable to allow extra time for the first assessment, as there is usually a long and complicated history, with symptoms involving many different areas.

The main complaint is pain, often widespread, diffuse and longstanding, going back from a few months to several years. One study found the duration of musculoskeletal complaints associated with JHS to range from 15 days to 45 years (El-Shahaly and El-Sherif 1991). There may be other symptoms, including stiffness (Kirk et al. 1967), clicking, clunking, subluxations, paraesthesiae, and some rather more bizarre symptoms, such as feeling 'like a bag of fleas' (personal communication).

These widespread symptoms often do not fit with how the patient looks or moves (Russek 2000), and in addition they may also report feeling unwell, suffering flu-like symptoms, feeling faint and being particularly tired. It is worth asking about other areas, as they may not volunteer information for fear of sounding like a hypochondriac

(Russek 2000, Lewkonia and Ansell 1983). Getting the complete picture not only helps with the diagnosis but gives the patient confidence that someone is really listening to them. It is helpful to let the patient talk, with the physiotherapist trying to resist the temptation to be too closed in their questioning. A lot of very useful information can be gained which will be helpful in piecing together the jigsaw puzzle.

Acasuso-Diaz et al. (1993) found that hypermobile individuals are more liable to develop musculoskeletal lesions. Pain is frequently reported at many sites, most commonly associated with joints (Kirk et al. 1967), and these individuals could be described as 'jointy' people (Maitland 1986). Knee pain was the most frequent complaint in the studies by Kirk et al. (1967) and El-Shahaly and El-Sherif (1991). Other frequently affected joints include the lumbar spine, shoulder, hands and wrists, cervical spine and ankles. Extra-articular soft tissue complaints are also reported as occurring frequently in hypermobile patients (El-Shahaly and El-Sherif 1991, Hudson et al. 1998), and take the form of tenosynovitis, tendonitis, bursitis, fasciitis and regional pain syndromes. Figure 6.3 illustrates a typical presentation.

Aggravating and easing factors in relation to pain are often not clearcut. Latency is a major factor, with the patient often reporting that an everyday activity can produce pain the next day or even the day after. This means it is often difficult to assess what the effect of the physical examination and treatment will be. Depending on the presentation, it may be advisable to do the minimum amount of examination necessary to make a clinical diagnosis and formulate a treatment plan, without treatment on the first attendance in order to prevent an exacerbation. Careful questioning regarding their response to physical activity will help the therapist to decide on how much to do in the examination. This careful approach often pays dividends, because the patient will have more confidence in the physiotherapist if there is no significant exacerbation following the examination.

In common with many joint problems, patients with JHS will report that they do not like sustained postures such as standing or sitting for prolonged periods. However, in this group of patients symptoms may well come on sooner than in non-hypermobile patients. Larsson et al. (1995) found that hypermobility of the spine caused an increased prevalence of back pain for industrial workers who worked in a standing or a sitting position. Similarly, hypermobility of the knees and spine was considered a liability, producing symptoms in musicians because of sustained standing postures (Larsson et al. 1993).

At the other end of the scale JHS patients also tolerate excessive or repetitive activity badly. They often tend to suffer symptoms after the activity rather than during it (Kirk et al. 1967), and it can be as long as 24–48 hours after the event. The symptoms are similar to a soft tissue strain, although there are frequently no signs of inflammation. Patients are often unable to recall a reason for the onset of symptoms, partly as the symptoms come on some time after the event, and because it may be that a normal everyday activity performed for slightly longer than usual or in slightly different circumstances is the culprit. This can be frustrating for physiotherapist and patient alike. Sometimes it is necessary to accept that it is not always possible to identify a cause for the symptoms, but gaining a clear understanding, through careful questioning, of how the symptoms of the syndrome affect the patient on a day-to-day basis is helpful. Patients vary tremendously, but many have pain on a daily basis. Some, in particular women with young children, often carry on regardless, feeling that they are unable to slow down or do less, and can reach a stage where their symptoms are such that they feel unable to cope. Others may reach a stage where they start restricting their activities to such an extent that they go into a downward spiral, with marked deconditioning and lack of confidence. Clinical depression is never far away. Both situations can have profoundly deleterious effects on their or their family's quality of life.

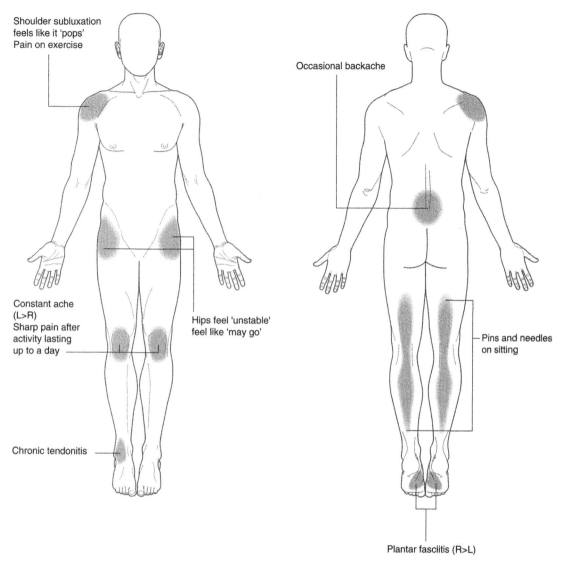

Figure 6.3 Typical symptoms in a JHS patient

Stiffness is a frequently reported symptom, with some complaining that they 'feel like a 90-year-old' when getting up in the morning. This subjective feeling of stiffness is often at odds with their range of movement on examination. Although their range of movement may look normal to the physiotherapist, questioning frequently reveals that it is restricted in comparison to the patient's normal range of movement. This is seen particularly in the middle-aged patient who has lost much of their former mobility. In the older patient, stiffness may be due to a general decrease in mobility with age (Seow et al. 1999), or secondary to joint injury or osteoarthritis. It is worth asking the patient if they were more flexible when younger, and a question such as 'have you ever been able to touch the floor with your palms flat' (Oliver 2000) often gives a clue to their previous flexibility and possible hypermobility. In addition, it may be helpful to ask whether they did ballet or gymnastics, as less flexible children do not usually do well in these activities. The importance of historical hypermobility has been acknowledged in the revised Brighton Criteria (Grahame et al. 2000), which in combination with other criteria can help with a diagnosis of JHS.

Hypermobile people often describe themselves as uncomfortable or fussy people who are constantly fidgeting and trying to get into a comfortable position (Oliver 2000). Russek (2000) describes a patient who complained of pain from where her body contacted the bed, and that this was relieved by using a thick feather comforter. This aspect of the hypermobility syndrome is reminiscent of the story of the Princess and the Pea, and perhaps suggests she was also a sufferer.

JHS is a heritable disorder and, on questioning, the patient may tell you that siblings, children or parents are similarly affected. Biro (1983) found that 27% of his cohort of patients had other family members with hypermobility, and Bridges et al. (1992) and Finsterbush and Pogrund (1982) found that 65% of their patients had first-degree relatives with a history of joint hypermobility. If a patient is unable to identify whether their relatives are hypermobile, it is worth asking if any of their relatives were gymnasts or dancers, or suffered from any joint problems. This will often reveal that a family member has had many diffuse chronic joint problems over the years, often having been given many diagnoses, such as osteoarthritis, spondylosis or disc prolapse without the symptoms being identified as due to JHS. Russek (2000) gives a good illustration of this.

Associated problems

As the hypermobility syndrome affects collagenous tissue there can be associated problems in other body systems. It is worth asking about other areas with this in mind. The presence of some of these can help to confirm the diagnosis.

There is evidence to suggest that uterine prolapse (El-Shahaly and El-Sherif 1991, Al-Rawi and Al-Rawi 1982) and abdominal hernias (Wynne-Davies 1971) are more common in JHS. Norton et al. (1995) found a significantly higher frequency of cystocele ($P = 0.001$), rectocele ($P = 0.0002$) and uterine prolapse ($P = 0.0002$) in women with hypermobility than in non-hypermobile women. Interestingly, there was no increased prevalence of stress incontinence in the hypermobile women. Tincello et al. (2002) likewise found that hypermobility was not associated with urinary incontinence, except that elbow hyperextension was associated with an increased incidence of postnatal urinary incontinence.

Patients report that they bruise very easily, noticing a bruise when they have no recollection of knocking themselves. Pitcher and Grahame (1982), Bulbena (1992), Bridges et al. (1992) and Kaplinsky et al. (1998) all report that easy bruising can be a feature of the hypermobility syndrome.

It has been suggested that patients with hypermobile joints often have laxity involving blood vessels (Bird and Barton 1993), and an increased incidence of varicose veins has been reported by El-Shahaly and El-Sherif (1991). There is also a possible association with Raynaud's phenomenon, as this has been reported as being more prevalent in a hypermobile group (Al-Rawi et al. 1985, El-Garf et al. 1998).

The presence of neuropathies has also been associated with hypermobility. Francis et al. (1987) report that nine out of 11 consecutive patients with tarsal tunnel syndrome were identified as having generalized hypermobility, and March et al. (1988) report on three patients in whom carpal tunnel syndrome was due to unusual sleep postures enabled by their joint hypermobility. They make the comment that identification of joint hypermobility and early management may mean that surgery is not needed in many cases.

Previous history

Previous injury can give an indication of how often and how easily a patient has injured themselves in the past. Hudson et al. (1998) found that hypermobile patients presenting to a rheumatology clinic were found to have significantly more previous episodes of soft tissue rheumatism (STR) and significantly more recurrent episodes at one site than non-hypermobile patients. This study also suggests that repetitive activity may be a contributing factor to the development of symptoms in some hypermobile individuals. Details of the type of activity the patient is regularly performing will help to identify possible mechanisms of injury and help in future management to prevent recurrences. A history of previous joint and soft tissue injury, in addition to indicating a possible diagnosis of JHS, will also give an indication of the speed of healing, which tends to be slower in these patients (Russek 2000).

Joint dislocations and subluxations are more common in people with hypermobility (Finsterbush and Pogrund, 1982). Spontaneous relocation usually occurs, particularly after the first time. Subsequent dislocations and subluxations often occur with no trauma, and some individuals can sublux and relocate a joint at will with little discomfort. The literature suggests the shoulder and patella to be the most frequently affected in adults (Beighton et al. 1989).

A history of pain in childhood or adolescence may be a further clue to the diagnosis of JHS. Pain in the knee, foot, ankle and back appears to be the most common, in descending order. The patient may also have complained of growing pains and delayed walking. This aspect is discussed in more detail in Chapter 4.

Patients frequently report that manual therapy has made them worse, or at best has failed to help. This is a useful piece of information, not only as a clue to a possible diagnosis of JHS, but also to ensure that similar techniques are not used again. It is unclear why manual therapy may aggravate the symptoms of JHS, but failing to recognize hypermobility and performing techniques too vigorously could be one explanation.

Box 6.1 gives a list of additional questions to ask during the subjective examination which can help in diagnosing JHS.

Box 6.1 Examples of additional questions that can be used to aid recognition of JHS

Previous history
Did they have pain as a child?
Did they have growing pains?
Did they do gymnastics or ballet when younger?
Were they more flexible when younger?
Did they feel better/worse in pregnancy?
Have they had any dislocations/subluxations?
Have they had many fractures?
How have they responded to analgesia?

Present history
Is there a family history of increased flexibility?
Do they dislike sustained postures, such as standing, sitting?
Do they dislike too much activity?
Do they bruise easily?
Do they have any herniae, varicose veins or prolapses?
Are they uncomfortable or fussy people?
Do they have any neuropathies?
Do they have Raynaud's phenomenon?

Physical examination

Observation

Observation starts from the moment a patient walks into the room. Clues that may lead the physiotherapist to begin to suspect JHS are the position the patient chooses to sit in the chair, and the movement of their hands. As previously mentioned, hypermobile patients often fidget and do not sit in one position for very long. They also often choose to sit in awkward positions, such as with one leg wrapped around the chair leg, or to side sit (Oliver 2000). This appears to be in an attempt to find more stability, using end-of-range positions, relying on tension in their ligaments, rather than resting in a neutral, midrange position where there is more movement and less stability. They frequently use their hands in an expressive way when talking, and increased mobility can often be observed in the metacarpal or interphalangeal joints (Fig. 6.4).

Skin can be thinner, stretchier and subject to striae, which are not due to a large weight change (Child 1986, Grahame 1989). Striae can often be seen at the base of the spine, around the thighs, shoulders and knees. Scar formation is often papyraceous or tissue-paper thin, and it is worth

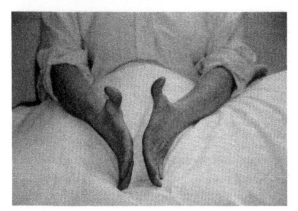

Figure 6.4 Hypermobility in the hands

looking at injection sites, childhood scars or surgery scars to assess tissue healing.

Muscle bulk may be decreased in certain muscles and hypermobile patients frequently have a lower muscle tone. Kirk et al. (1967) noted that several of their group of hypermobile patients had poor muscular development.

Static posture

Flat feet are associated with hypermobility (El-Garf et al. 1998, Al-Rawi et al. 1985) and have been reported as being present in 85% of hypermobile patients referred to a rheumatologist (Bridges et al. 1992). This should be assessed in a static posture and in walking. Some hypermobile individuals can appear to have good medial arches but which collapse on weight bearing. Loss of the medial arch will have an effect on the alignment and dynamics of the lower limbs. In addition, hallux abducto valgus has also been shown to be associated with hypermobility (Harris and Beeson 1998).

An assessment of posture in standing, from all directions and involving the whole body, is made and compared to the standard posture. The standard posture is one that demonstrates maximal efficiency and involves the minimum amount of stress and strain on the body (Kendall et al. 1993). It is seen when there are normal spinal curves, ideal alignment of the lower limbs for weight bearing, and the muscle system is in

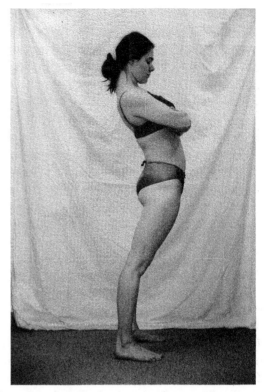

Figure 6.5 Sway-back posture in a hypermobile patient

balance. Hypermobile patients frequently demonstrate a sway-back or a kyphosis–lordosis posture, as described by Kendall et al. (1993).

Postural alignment in hypermobile patients frequently exhibits an attempt to gain more stability through resting at the end of range of hypermobile joints. There is frequently hyperextension at the knees and patients can be seen to rest at the end of their range, which may be up to an extra 25°. This can be associated with a compensatory hyperextension in the hips, which produces a forward displacement of the pelvis so that the weight is taken forward over the feet. This sway forward usually leads to a compensatory increase in the thoracic kyphosis and a flattening of the lumbar spine (Kendall et al. 1993). The hypermobile patient shown in Figure 6.5 is showing a sway-back posture, resting at the end of range of extension at the hips and knees, with a forward displacement of the pelvis. It is easy to see that this patient is potentially stressing her

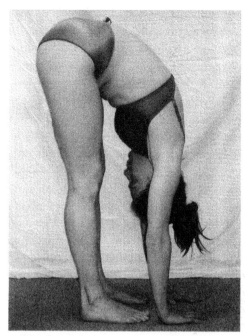

Figure 6.6   Spinal flexion in a hypermobile patient

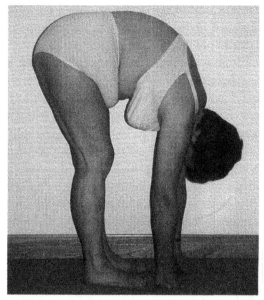

Figure 6.7   Increased thoracic spinal flexion during forward spinal flexion

knees, hips and lumbar spine by adopting this posture and, not surprisingly, complains of pain in her back and hips. Hypermobile patients frequently demonstrate poor neck posture, with the head held forward with overactive upper trapezius muscles.

Active movement testing

The active range of movement often looks normal, but the important question is, is it normal for them? Their mobility may appear normal and hence not fit with their reports of stiffness. Further questioning of the patient will help to clarify these points.

It is often not possible to reproduce 'their' pain on examination, and if some pain is produced it often does not fit with their pain description. This is most likely because generally it is not movement alone that produces pain in a hypermobile patient but rather sustained postures, or continuing a particular movement for a prolonged period. In view of the observation and reports that pain can take 48 hours to come on after an activity, it is unwise to subject the patient

to extensive testing of their mobility, in terms of either repeated testing or vigorous overpressure. It pays to rely on their subjective feelings during testing, and if overpressure is required to gain further information this should be done gently to give an idea of end feel, rather than to stress the joint(s) at the end of range.

When testing range of movement it is important to look at the range achieved, but as their symptoms may not be reproduced, it is essential that the quality of the movement is observed. Hypermobile patients frequently demonstrate the ability to touch their ankles or feet when bending forwards and report no discomfort or reproduction of symptoms except a feeling of stiffness. This is because their normal range is to easily place their palms flat on the floor in this position (Fig. 6.6), and even though the movement looks normal for non-hypermobile patients it is not normal for them. It is important to assess where the movement is occurring. Forward bending or flexion of the spine may show increased hip flexion and increased length of hamstrings but poor lumbar spine flexion. They may show increased thoracic flexion (Fig. 6.7) with a flat, relatively immobile lumbar spine. It is therefore important to identify areas of relative hypermobility and relative hypomobility.

In spinal extension there is frequently an increased range of movement in the mid or low lumbar spine and virtually no movement in the thoracic spine. There may be evidence of hinging occurring at a particular level, where the movement is seen to be excessive rather than occurring in a smooth curve (Fig. 6.8). This suggests hypermobility or functional instability at this level, and is frequently associated with pain. In these patients it appears that because they have hypermobility in the lumbar spine into extension and hence it is easier to move here, they get almost all their range in the lumbar spine and consequently stop using the thoracic spine when extending. Some of this may also be related to the increased sedentary nature of our lifestyle, which facilitates a slouching posture and hence an increased flexion of the

thoracic spine. Some individuals, when asked to bend backwards, can be observed to use hip extension, if there is increased range at the hip, in addition to or instead of lumbar spine movement.

Lateral flexion in the spine frequently demonstrates increased mobility, with the patient easily reaching 5–8 cm below the knee crease with their fingertips. A similar pattern is often seen in the cervical spine, where some hypermobile patients can put their ear on their shoulder. Rotation in the cervical spine is often hypermobile, showing a range of over 90°, with the chin reaching level with or just beyond the shoulder. Extension is frequently of good range without symptoms, but often occurs in the upper and mid cervical spine, with minimal or no movement in the low cervical or upper thoracic spine.

Observing how the patient moves when walking, from sitting to standing, or when doing an activity that produces symptoms, is necessary to identify where movement is occurring. Here again, it is helpful to identify areas of relative hyper- and hypomobility. There may be increased rotation of the lumbar spine, increased extension at the hip, over-pronation in the feet, increased medial rotation of the femur, and hyperextension at the knees. If symptoms are not produced, it is helpful to ask the patient to describe what they are feeling while doing these activities. They are often able to describe stiffness, uneven weight-bearing, or feelings of instability in various parts of their body with particular movements.

The 'stiffness' of which some hypermobile patients complain, and which is not related to restriction of active movement, may be related to the feeling of 'stiffness' relating to muscles. This is the resistance felt when a muscle is passively elongated. A hypertrophied muscle is stiffer than a weak or atrophied one. This 'stiffness' occurs through the range rather than at the end of range. It has been described as similar to the resistance felt when elongating a spring (Sahrmann 2002). Thixotrophy also contributes to muscle stiffness and may be why hypermobile patients report benefit from stretching.

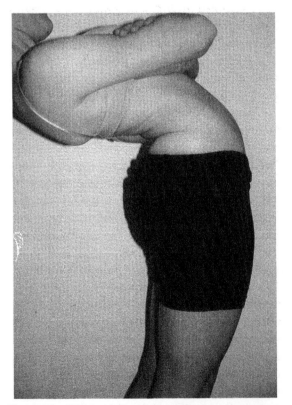

Figure 6.8 'Hinging' in the lumbar spine during extension

The patterns of movement that patients adopt during the assessment can give clues to likely muscle imbalances, which can be tested more fully. Considerations here are muscle strength, length, timing, and whether any compensatory movements are occurring, or compensatory relative flexibility as described by Sahrmann (2002). This concept is illustrated by imagining that the body is controlled by a series of springs. These vary in extensibility such that increased stiffness in one group can produce compensatory movement at adjoining areas, which are controlled by muscles which have less stiffness. An illustration of this can be seen in Figure 6.9. On testing knee flexion in prone, compensatory movement is seen to occur in the form of an increase in lumbar extension and anterior pelvic tilt (Fig. 6.9b). This is not due to shortness in the rectus femoris muscles, as when the pelvis is stabilized by the physiotherapist the knee is still able to flex to full range (Fig. 6.9c). Movement in the spine is compensatory, resulting from increased or excessive flexibility into the direction of extension compared to the relative stiffness in the rectus femoris muscle.

Compensatory movement can also occur as a result of poor motor control and altered recruitment patterns. Hypermobile patients frequently show increased flexibility into wrist flexion during finger extension (Fig. 6.10). The wrist flexors, which should contract to prevent wrist extension and keep the wrist in neutral, actually produce movement into flexion. This can result in a reduction of the carpal tunnel space and may lead to carpal tunnel syndrome (Sahrmann 2002).

Observation of poor muscle bulk may indicate muscle weakness, which can be confirmed by testing muscle strength. For example, a person who stands in a sway posture is likely to have decreased gluteal bulk and tone and gluteus maximus tests weak. Muscles that are habitually held in an elongated position can also become weak, such as the one-joint hip flexors, in a person who habitually stands in hip extension.

Measuring hypermobility

The various scoring systems for measuring hypermobility in current use (Beighton, Contompasis, Bulbena etc.) are covered in Chapter 1.

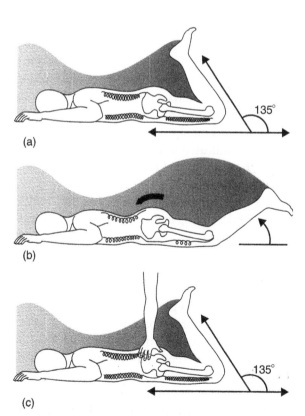

(a)

(b)

(c)

Figure 6.9 Compensatory lumbopelvic motion during knee flexion associated with differences in the stiffness of the abdominal and rectus femoris muscles. (From Sahrmann (2002), with permission.)

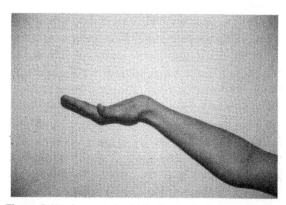

Figure 6.10 Increased wrist flexion during finger extension

The Beighton scale is quick and easy to use to confirm hypermobility in the clinic, although there are criticisms of this scoring system. When examining a patient who is suspected of being hypermobile it is important to consider other joints not included in this scale, and the extent to which they move as well as movement in other planes. The shoulder is often found to be hypermobile, with many patients reaching 90° in horizontal extension, beyond 180° into elevation, beyond 85° lateral rotation in neutral and beyond 90° in 90° abduction. There is often increased rotation at the hips, particularly medial rotation, as well as increased abduction. The proximal and distal interphalangeal joints frequently hyperextend. In addition, Bulbena et al. (1992) found that excessive ankle dorsiflexion and foot eversion were the most common characteristics in a group of hypermobile subjects, being present in 94%, and patellar hypermobility was found to be present in 89%. First metatarsophalangeal extension beyond 90° is also commonly found.

The Beighton scale can also fail to confirm a diagnosis of hypermobility in the older patient whose range of movement has decreased with age. Hypermobility of the trunk was found in younger patients (average age 37 years) but not in the older group of hypermobile patients (average age 62 years) (Bridges et al. 1992).

Passive movement testing

Passive movement testing can be helpful in confirming hypermobility, although caution should be applied as these tests may exacerbate symptoms. Hypermobile joints frequently feel 'freer' or 'looser' than non-hypermobile joints, with less resistance being encountered throughout the range. The neutral zone (Panjabi 1992b) is larger than in non-hypermobile joints. When resistance is encountered it tends to occur suddenly towards the end of the movement, and the end-feel is usually softer than in non-hypermobile joints. The end-feel – the sensation felt by the examiner's hand at the end of range of hypermobile joints – has been described as having an empty, 'boggy' or 'soggy' quality. When resistance is encountered it is often hard and springy, suggesting muscle spasm rather than a restriction due to tight or fibrosed tissue.

Extra care is needed in handling hypermobile joints and tissues. JHS patients have a tendency towards increased fragility and vulnerability in their collagenous tissues. In addition, the latent nature of the pain means that it is difficult to know when strain, sufficient to produce symptoms, is being put on the tissues until it is too late. During all passive handling of hypermobile tissues it is necessary for the physiotherapist to pay attention to how the joint and tissues feel and behave in their hands during movement. It is advisable not to push too hard into the end of range, particularly if there is a soft end-feel.

Particular care should be taken with the vertebral artery and upper cervical spine ligament testing. It can be argued that it is unnecessary and possibly dangerous to do these tests on a hypermobile neck. Both tests involve stressing the end of range, and consequently the ligaments and soft tissues in the cervical spine. As it is unlikely that a manipulation of the cervical spine would be indicated or appropriate in the hypermobile patient, for the most part, it is advisable to exclude these tests.

Care is also needed with neural mobility testing (Butler 1991). Testing in the upper and lower limbs frequently needs to be taken further because of the increase in range of movement. However, it can be very easy to over-stretch. Testing procedures should be performed slowly, with attention to the feel of the tissues. Hypermobile patients frequently have a large amplitude of movement with virtually no resistance present. Resistance comes in quickly towards the end of the movement and may be encountered before any symptoms. It is wise to stop testing at this point to prevent an exacerbation. Paraesthesiae affecting the hands, feet or both are reported frequently by hypermobile patients (El-Shahaly and El-Sherif 1991), and are often reproduced on testing neural mobility.

Palpation

Not all the joints in a JHS patient are necessarily hypermobile. Some areas, such as the thoracic spine and cervicothoracic junction, have a tendency to stiffen. This may be one reason for some of the bizarre symptoms reported which are being mediated via the sympathetic nervous system. These stiff areas have the potential to increase stress on the hypermobile sections in the spine, commonly the midcervical and lumbar spine, which may be responsible for symptoms. Palpation findings should confirm what has been observed during movement testing.

During passive movement testing it is important to ensure that movement is taking place where it is intended to take place. When palpating a stiff joint in the spine it is possible to produce symptoms at another area of the spine some distance from the one being palpated. This is because the pressure normally exerted to produce movement at the stiff area is producing strain further away. It is important in this instance to observe the whole spine, pay careful attention to what is being felt, and support hypermobile sections when necessary. For example, palpation of a stiff thoracic spine in the prone position will place less stress on the lumbar spine if a pillow is used to lift the lumbar spine out of extension.

WOMEN'S HEALTH

As generalized joint hypermobility and JHS are reported to occur more frequently in females it is appropriate to consider issues that affect women.

There have been some potential risks in pregnancy reported in women with joint hypermobility. Thornton et al. (1988) report on two generations of women affected by JHS where pregnancies were complicated by unexplained midtrimester vaginal bleeding. Severe prematurity, due to cervical incompetence and premature rupture of the membranes, has been reported in a patient with the hypermobility type of EDS (DeVos et al. 1999), and Charvet et al. (1991), in a

literature review, report similar occurrences in addition to tears and perineal haematomas. It is important that physiotherapists are aware of these potential complications, particularly if the patient has not previously been identified as hypermobile. It may well be appropriate to have the diagnosis confirmed by a rheumatologist so that the obstetrician can be informed of these potential problems.

Hypermobile women often report a considerable change in their feeling of wellbeing during pregnancy. For some asymptomatic individuals it seems that pregnancy was the start of their problems and that they have been symptomatic ever since. Others report that they felt the best they have ever felt, or even became symptom free for the first time in years while pregnant, only to have all their symptoms return soon after delivery.

The literature suggests that around 50% of women suffer back or posterior pelvic pain while pregnant (Ostgaard et al. 1993). The reason for the high prevalence of spinal pain associated with pregnancy is not known. Several hypotheses have been put forward, but no one factor has been found to be responsible. It is likely that the cause is multifactorial, although increased mobility of the pelvic joints due to hormonal changes affecting the ligaments has been found to play a part, and may be particularly relevant in the JHS patient.

Research in this area divides spinal pain associated with pregnancy into two distinct areas: back pain (lumbar spine) and peripartum pelvic pain (PPPP) (pain in the pelvic region) (Mens et al. 1996). PPPP has been found to be four times as common as back pain during pregnancy, and although fitness prior to pregnancy reduces the incidence of back pain in pregnancy, it was found to make no difference to PPPP (Ostgaard et al. 1994). It has been suggested that the increased laxity of ligaments due to hormonal changes may be responsible, with higher concentrations of relaxin being found in pregnant women with PPPP than in controls (MacLennan et al. 1986).

Ligament laxity was found to increase throughout pregnancy, particularly from the 12th to the

20th week (Ostgaard et al. 1993), and therefore the stability of the pelvis may be affected long before any significant weight gain has occurred. In addition, the study by Ostgaard et al. (1993) found that the increase in peripheral laxity in the primiparous pregnant group took 36 weeks to reach the same level as the multipregnant group reached at 12 weeks. This suggests that the increased peripheral laxity associated with pregnancy does not return to its prepregnancy level. This may have consequences for the hypermobile patient in terms of further pregnancies, but may also help to explain why for many hypermobile women their symptoms start with the first pregnancy and do not disappear after delivery. In addition, Frank et al. (personal communication), found generalized hypermobility to be the only significant predictor of postpartum spinal pain.

Ostgaard et al. (1993) found that a large sagittal diameter of the abdomen correlated weakly with back pain in pregnancy, but strongly with peripheral laxity. They suggest that women with high peripheral laxity may develop larger abdomens owing to an increase in extensibility of the abdominal wall. This is due to collagen insufficiency caused by the hormones. This increases the flexion moment on the back and may increase the risk of back pain. Back pain did not correlate with laxity in multiparous women, but did correlate with laxity in primiparous women in the 12th week. They conclude that an increase in collagen laxity would result in less ability to resist stretching, and may indicate a minor risk factor for back pain in pregnant women.

It is not known what influence pregnancy has on generalized joint hypermobility. Although there is evidence that mobility in peripheral joints increases significantly during pregnancy (Calguneri et al. 1982, Ostgaard et al. 1993), the study by Calguneri et al. (1982) showed no change in the Beighton score. This is probably due to a lack of sensitivity inherent in the scale. In women who are already affected by generalized joint hypermobility, pregnancy could make them unstable in certain areas, particularly the pelvis, causing symptoms. There is no evidence at present that hypermobile women have an increased occurrence of back pain during pregnancy or PPPP because of increased mobility. To the author's knowledge the only research that has addressed this issue is by van Dongen et al. (1999). This study examined hypermobility and PPPP in 509 Cape Coloured pregnant women. Although they found no correlation between hypermobility and PPPP, they comment that PPPP was virtually absent in this group and that hypermobility was surprisingly low, at 5%. It is therefore difficult to draw any conclusions from this study, and further research in this area is clearly needed.

In spite of not knowing what effects generalized hypermobility may have in pregnancy it is helpful to review what is known about the presentation of PPPP in pregnant women, insofar as it is related to joint laxity.

Women with PPPP usually present with pain around the sacroiliac joints, symphysis pubis, buttocks and upper legs. Pain is related to weight-bearing, such that standing and walking provoke pain (Ostgaard 1998), and many patients show a characteristic waddling gait (Mens et al. 1996), with or without a marked limp on one side. The pain is time-dependent, with the patient being able to do most of what she used to do, but for a shorter time. The pain, when provoked by overdoing things, will often be felt the following day rather than immediately, and this sounds remarkably similar to the onset of pain reported by JHS patients. Twisting and asymmetric loading of the pelvis, as in vacuum cleaning, is most painful (Ostgaard 1998). The posterior pelvic pain provocation test (Ostgaard 1998), developed to differentiate women with pelvic pain rather than back pain, is positive. The test constitutes a gentle longitudinal pressure applied along the femur with the hip in 90° flexion and the patient supine. The test is positive if pain is produced in the posterior pelvis on the examined side only (Ostgaard 1998). PPPP is thought to be due to

Case study

A 36-year-old man was referred for physiotherapy in connection with a series of musculoskeletal complaints in the presence of joint hypermobility. He was normally fit, exercising regularly, running, playing water polo and swimming competitively until 2 years prior to referral. He had had no problems as a child, although he had dislocated his left elbow at the age of 17.

His problems started 4 years earlier, when he suffered left knee pain and a feeling as if the joint had 'given out' after a walk down a mountain. This settled, but pain returned after he started running 2 years later. He stopped running and diagnosed a tight iliotibial band (ITB) as the cause, and treated this himself with stretches. The pain continued, settling into a fairly constant ache with a sharp pain on activity, such as walking uphill, which could take a day or two to subside. He was still unable to run. In the meantime he had also injured his right ankle snowboarding, and this was diagnosed as a chronic strain or tendonitis.

Six months prior to referral, he subluxed his right shoulder while swimming. This relocated spontaneously but left him with some discomfort, which increased when doing arm exercises with weights at the gym. He was diagnosed with an impingement syndrome and referred for physiotherapy, which was unhelpful. At around this time he also developed right knee pain, bilateral plantar fasciitis, and a feeling of his hips being unstable. He describes this as a period when his 'whole body went'. He stopped all physical activity, but this had no beneficial effect on his symptoms: in fact he felt they were all deteriorating. He reported feeling 'as if he was 100 years old' in the morning, feeling stiff and shuffling for an hour after rising. His pain chart at the time of assessment is illustrated in Figure 6.3.

He was in good health, although his weight had increased because of the lack of exercise. He was in a sedentary desk job. Non-steroidal anti-inflammatory medication had not been helpful. He had seen various medical practitioners before seeing a rheumatologist, who recognized his generalized hypermobility and referred him to our clinic. His blood tests were negative and X-rays and scans had shown mild degenerative changes in the left patella only.

On examination he stood in a sway posture, with flat feet, hyperextended knees and an increased thoracic kyphosis. He had a forward head posture and his shoulders were forward with the scapulae abducted (right > left). He had decreased gluteal bulk and slight wasting of the quadriceps on the left. Muscle tone was decreased generally over much of his body. The range and quality of spinal mobility were good. He could reach the floor with his fingers on bending forward, and showed some increased flexibility in the lumbar spine into extension and some stiffness in the thoracic spine. He scored 4/9 on the Beighton score (5/9 historically), and outside the scale he showed increased mobility in his hips into lateral rotation and abduction and his shoulders into elevation and external rotation.

He demonstrated poor trunk stability, with overactivity of the external oblique muscle. There was muscle imbalance around the hips, with shortness of ITB and dominance of the hamstrings over gluteus maximus. The gluteal muscles tested weak. There was a painful arc in the right shoulder and tenderness on palpation of supraspinatus. The upper fibres of trapezius were overactive, with weak lower trapezius producing poor stabilization of the scapulae during movement. The patellofemoral joint showed lateral tracking (left worse than right), with some associated tilt.

The impression from the examination was that this hypermobile man experienced no symptoms while he was physically fit and strong. An unresolved knee problem, which started after unaccustomed activity and a strain to the ankle, set in motion compensatory mechanisms to protect the joints, and a gradual decrease in physical exercise eventually resulted in further joint problems and a cessation of all exercise, resulting in the patient becoming deconditioned and weaker.

---

laxity of the ligaments and capsule of the sacroiliac joints owing to certain hormones, leading to instability through inadequate force closure (Pool-Goudzwaard et al. 1998). Hip and spinal movements are full and, interestingly, Ostgaard (1998) remarks that often these women can easily reach the floor with straight knees, which may suggest that generalized hypermobility is a factor in the development of this condition and that hyper-mobile women may be more at risk of suffering PPPP.

CONCLUSION

Generalized joint hypermobility is frequently the cause of musculoskeletal symptoms reported by patients consulting physiotherapists. The condition is often misunderstood and underrecognized. Gaining a better understanding of how the complaint presents and affects the JHS patient will help the physiotherapist recognize the condition and aid assessment and management.

REFERENCES

Acasuso-Diaz, M., Collantes-Estevez, E. and Sánchez Guijo, P. (1993) Joint hyperlaxity and musculoligamentous lesions: study of a population of homogeneous age, sex and physical exertion. *British Journal of Rheumatology*, **32**, 120–2.

Al-Rawi, Z.S. and Al-Rawi, Z.T. (1982) Joint hypermobility in women with genital prolapse. *Lancet*, **1**, 1439–41.

Al-Rawi, Z.S., Al-Aszawi, A.J. and Al-Chalabi, T. (1985) Joint mobility among university students in Iraq. *British Journal of Rheumatology*, **4**, 326–31.

Al-Rawi, Z. and Nessan, A.H. (1997) Joint hypermobility in patients with chondromalacia patellae. *British Journal of Rheumatology*, **12**, 1324–7.

Barton, L.M. and Bird, H.A. (1996) Improving pain by the stabilization of hyperlax joints. *Journal of Ortho Rheumatology*, **9**, 46–51.

Beighton, P., Grahame, R. and Bird, H. (1989) Hypermobility of joints, 2nd edn. Springer-Verlag.

Beighton, P., Grahame, R. and Bird, H. (1999) Hypermobility of joints, 3rd edn, p 130. Springer-Verlag.

Bergmark, A. (1989) Stability of the lumbar spine. A study in mechanical engineering. *Acta Orthopedica Scandinavica*, **230** (Suppl), 20–4.

Bird, H.A. and Barton, L. (1993) Joint hyperlaxity and its long term effect on joints. *Journal of the Royal Society of Health*, December, 327–9.

Bird, H.A., Tribe, C R. and Bacon, P.A. (1978) Joint hypermobility leading to osteoarthritis and chondrocalcinosis. *Annals of the Rheumatic Diseases*, **37**, 203–11.

Biro, F., Gewanter, H.L. and Baum, J. (1983) The hypermobility syndrome. *Pediatrics*, **72**, 701–6.

Bridges, A.J., Smith, E. and Reid, J. (1992) Joint hypermobility in adults referred to rheumatology clinics. *Annals of the Rheumatic Diseases*, **51**, 793–6.

Bulbena, A., Duro, J.C., Porta, M. et al. (1992) Clinical assessment of hypermobility of joints: assembling criteria. *Journal of Rheumatology*, **19**, 115–22.

Butler, D.S. (1991) *Mobilisation of the Nervous System*. Churchill Livingstone.

Calguneri, M., Bird, H. and Wright, V. (1982) Changes in joint laxity during pregnancy. *Annals of the Rheumatic Diseases*, **41**, 126–8.

Charvet, P.Y., Salle, B., Rebaud, P. et al. (1991) [Ehlers–Danlos syndrome and pregnancy. Apropos of a case] [Abstract – article in French]. *Journal of Gynecology Biology and Reproduction (Paris)*, **20**, 75–8.

Cherpel, A. and Marks, R. (1999) The benign joint hypermobility syndrome. *New Zealand Journal of Physiotherapy*, **27**, 9–22.

Child, A.H. (1986) Joint hypermobility syndrome: inherited disorder of collagen synthesis. *Journal of Rheumatology*, **13**, 239–43.

De Vos, M., Nuytinck, L., Verellen, C. and De Paepe, A. (1999) Preterm premature rupture of membranes in a patient with the hypermobility type of the Ehlers–Danlos syndrome. A case report. *Fetal Diagnostics and Therapy*, **14**, 244–7.

El-Garf, A.K., Mahmoud, G.A. and Mahgoub, E.H. (1998) Hypermobility among Egyptian children: prevalence and features. *Journal of Rheumatology*, **5**, 1003–5.

El-Shahaly, H.A. and El-Sherif, A.K. (1991) Is the benign hypermobility syndrome benign? *Clinical Rheumatology*, **10**, 302–7.

Finsterbush, A. and Pogrund, H. (1982) The hypermobility syndrome. Musculoskeletal complaints in 100 consecutive cases of generalized joint hypermobility. *Clinical Orthopedics*, **168**, 124–7.

Francis, H., March, L., Terenty, T. and Webb, J. (1987) Benign joint hypermobility with neuropathy: documentation of tarsal tunnel syndrome. *Journal of Rheumatology*, **14**, 577–81.

Gannon, L.M. and Bird, H.A. (1999) The quantification of joint laxity in dancers and gymnasts. *Journal of Sports Science*, **9**, 743–50.

Gazit, Y., Nahir, A.M., Grahame, R. and Jacob, G. (2003) Dysautonomia in the joint hypermobility syndrome. *American Journal of Medicine*, **115**, 33–40.

Grahame, R. (1986) Clinical manifestations of the joint hypermobility syndrome. *Reumatologia (USSR)*, **2**, 20–4.

Grahame, R. (1989) Clinical conundrum. How often, when and how does joint hypermobility lead to osteoarthritis? *British Journal of Rheumatology*, **28**, 320.

Grahame, R. (1999) Joint hypermobility and genetic collagen disorders: are they related? *Archives of Disease in Childhood*, **80**, 188–91.

Grahame, R. (2000) Heritable disorders of connective tissue. In *Baillière's Best Practice and Research in Clinical Rheumatology* (Balint and Bardin, eds), Vol. 14(2), pp. 345–361.

Grahame, R., Bird, H.A., Child, A. et al. (2000) The Revised (Brighton 1998) criteria for the Diagnosis of Benign Hypermobility Syndrome (BJHS). *Journal of Rheumatology*, **27**, 1777–9.

Harris, M.-C.R. and Beeson, P. (1998) Generalized hypermobility: is it a predisposing factor towards the development of juvenile hallux abducto valgus. *The Foot*, **8**, 203–9.

Hudson, N., Fitzcharles, M.-A., Cohen, M., Starr, M.R. and Esdaile, J.M. (1998) The association of soft tissue rheumatism and hypermobility. *British Journal of Rheumatology*, **37**, 382–6.

Jessee, E.F., Owen, D.S. and Sagar, K.B. (1980) The benign hypermobility syndrome. *Arthritis and Rheumatism*, **23**, 1053–6.

Kaplinsky, C., Kenet, G., Seligsohn, U. and Rechavi, G. (1998) Association between hyperflexibility of the thumb and an unexplained bleeding tendency: is it a rule of thumb? *British Journal of Haematology*, **101**, 260–3.

Kendall, F.P., McCreary, E.K. and Provance, P.G. (1993) *Muscles: Testing and Function*, 4th edn. Williams &Wilkins.

Kerr, A., Macmillan, C.E., Uttley, W.S. and Luqmani, R.A. (2000) Physiotherapy for children with hypermobility syndrome. *Physiotherapy*, **86**, 313–17.

Kirk, J.A., Ansell, B.M. and Bywaters, E.G.L. (1967) The hypermobility syndrome. Muscular complaints associated with generalized joint hypermobility. *Annals of the Rheumatic Diseases*, **26**, 419–25.

Larsson, L.G., Baum, J., Mudholker, G.S. and Kollia, G.D. (1993) Benefits and disadvantages of joint hypermobility among musicians. *New England Journal of Medicine*, **329**, 1079–82.

Larsson, L.G., Mudholker, G.S., Baum, J. and Srivastava, D.K. (1995) Benefits and liabilities of hypermobility in the back pain disorders of industrial workers. *Journal of Internal Medicine*, **5**, 461–7.

Lewkonia, R.M. and Ansell, B.M. (1983) Articular hypermobility simulating chronic rheumatic disease. *Archives of Disease in Childhood*, **12**, 988–92.

MacLennan, A.H., Nicholson, R., Green, R.C. et al. (1986) Serum relaxin and pelvic pain of pregnancy. *Lancet*, **ii**, 243–5.

Maitland, G.D. (1986) *Vertebral Manipulation*, 5th edn. Appendix 4, pp. 374. Butterworth Scientific.

March, L.M., Francis, H. and Webb, J. (1988) Benign joint hypermobility with neuropathies: documentation of median, sciatic and common peroneal nerve compression. *Clinical Rheumatology*, **7**, 35–40.

Mens, J.M.A., Vleeming, A., Stoeckart, R. et al. (1996) Understanding peripartum pelvic pain. Implications of a patient survey. *Spine*, **21**, 1363–70.

Norton, P.A., Baker, J.E., Sharp, H.C. and Warenski, J.C. (1995) Genitourinary prolapse and joint hypermobility in women. *Obstetrics and Gynecology*, **85**, 225–8.

Oliver, J. (2000) Hypermobility: recognition and management. *In Touch*, **94**, 9–12.

O'Sullivan, P.B. (2000) Lumbar segmental 'instability': clinical presentation and specific stabilizing exercise management. *Manual Therapy*, **5**, 2–12.

Ostgaard, H.C. (1998) Assessment and treatment of low back pain in working pregnant women. In: *Proceedings of the Third Interdisciplinary World Congress on Low Back Pain and Pelvic Pain* (A.Vleeming, V. Mooney, H. Tilscher et al. eds), pp. 161–71. Vienna, Austria.

Ostgaard, H.C., Andersson, G.B.J., Schultz, A.B. and Miller, J.A.A. (1993) Influence of some biomechanical factors on low-back pain in pregnancy. *Spine*, **18**, 61–5.

Ostgaard, H.C., Zetherstrom, G., Roos-Hansson, E. and Svanberg, B. (1994) Reduction of back and posterior pelvic pain in pregnancy. *Spine*, **19**, 894–900.

Panjabi, M.M. (1992a) The stabilizing system of the spine. Part I. Function, dysfunction, adaptation and enhancement. *Journal of Spinal Disorders*, **5**, 383–9.

Panjabi, M.M. (1992b) The stabilizing system of the spine. Part II. Neutral zone and instability hypothesis. *Journal of Spinal Disorders*, **5**, 390–7.

Pitcher, D. and Grahame, R. (1982) Mitral valve prolapse and joint hypermobility: evidence for a connective tissue abnormality? *Annals of the Rheumatic Diseases*, **4**, 352–4.

Pool-Goodzwaard, A.L., Vleeming, A., Stoeckart, R. et al. (1998) Insufficient lumbopelvic stability: a clinical, anatomical and biomechanical approach to 'a-specific' low back pain. *Manual Therapy*, **3**, 12–20.

Richardson, C., Jull, G., Hodges, P. and Hides, J. (1999) *Therapeutic Exercise for Spinal Segmental Stabilisation in Low Back Pain*. Churchill Livingstone.

Russek, L.N. (1999) Hypermobility syndrome. *Physical Therapy*, **79**, 591–9.

Russek, L.N. (2000) Examination and treatment of a patient with hypermobility syndrome. *Physical Therapy*, **80**, 386–98.

Sahrmann, S. (2002) *Diagnosis and Treatment of Movement Impairment Syndromes*. Mosby.

Seow, C.C., Chow, P.K. and Khong, K.S. (1999) A study of joint mobility in a normal population. *Annals of the Academy of Medicine of Singapore*, **2**, 231–6.

Thornton, J.G., Hill, J. and Bird, H.A. (1988) Complications of pregnancy and benign familial joint hyperlaxity. *Annals of the Rheumatic Diseases*, **47**, 228–31.

Tincello, A.G., Adams, E.J. and Richmond, D.H. (2002) Antenatal screening for postpartum urinary incontinence in nulliparous women: a pilot study. *European Journal of Obstetrics Gynecology and Reproductive Biology*, **1**, 70–3.

van Dongen, P.W., de Boer, M., Lemmens, W.A. and Theron, G.B. (1999) Hypermobility and peripartum pelvic pain syndrome in pregnant African women. *European Journal of Obstetrics Gynecology and Reproductive Biology*, **1**, 77–82.

Verhoeven, J.J., Tuinman, M. and Van Dongen, P.W. (1999) Joint hypermobility in African non-pregnant nulliparous women. *European Journal of Obstetrics Gynecology and Reproductive Biology*, **1**, 69–72.

Wordsworth, P., Ogilvie, D., Smith, R. and Sykes, B. (1987) Joint mobility with particular reference to racial variation and inherited connective tissue disorders. *British Journal of Rheumatology*, **1**, 9–12.

Wynne-Davies, R. (1971) Familial joint laxity. *Proceedings of the Royal Society of Medicine*, **64**, 689–90.

7

Management of the hypermobile adult

Rosemary Keer
Anna Edwards-Fowler
Elizabeth Mansi

Aims

1. To discuss the role of manual therapy and muscle re-education in the restoration of normal mobility and muscle balance with the aim of improving function and reducing disability
2. To highlight the importance of educating the patient about the condition, with guidelines to enable the physiotherapist to help patients to manage the problem effectively themselves
3. To discuss management of symptoms associated with pregnancy in hypermobile individuals
4. To provide suggestions to help the physiotherapist and patient solve many of the common problems presented by JHS

INTRODUCTION

There is little written in the physiotherapy literature about treatment in relation to JHS and even less on research into the efficacy of different treatment modalities. However, physiotherapists are experienced in the treatment and rehabilitation of joint laxity and instability due to ligament damage and degenerative joint diseases. It would seem logical, therefore, in the absence of proven treatment techniques or regimens, to apply the treatment principles used in these conditions to the management of JHS (Cherpel and Marks 1999). Once the hypermobility syndrome has been recognized it is possible to formulate a treatment plan, taking into account presenting signs and symptoms, previous history, the tendency to less robust tissues, increased flexibility, possible instability and increased healing time. It should take into account the whole person and include prognosis and advice to allow the patient to manage their problem effectively themselves. Although it is appropriate to treat acute episodes with physiotherapy, the main aim of treatment in this group of people is to increase function and reduce disability. This often involves reassurance and patient education, stability and muscle endurance work, and some activity and lifestyle modification.

Although the aim of treatment for JHS patients is diminished impairment and functional limitation it is likely that many hypermobile patients will have recurrent problems throughout their life (Russek 2000). The case study at the end of this chapter, and the one given by Russek (2000), both show that JHS patients with chronic diffuse widespread pain are likely to have continuing problems. However, with recognition of the condition and appropriate guidance the patient can learn to manage the problem more effectively, thereby reducing suffering and gaining a better quality of life.

The majority of patients complain of pain associated with the musculoskeletal system. Finsterbush and Pogrund (1982) identified several different pain groups in their study. One group had long-standing mild musculoskeletal complaints, a second group had acute episodes of pain at various sites, and the third group had features which were a combination of the first two. This would seem to be a reasonable description of the presentation of symptoms in the JHS patient, although in the authors' experience many suffer symptoms which are rather more than mild.

As yet it is not known why some hypermobile patients experience pain whereas others do not. However, the hypothesis that pain is caused by microtrauma to tissues from overuse or misuse of hypermobile joints, would appear to explain part of the mechanism. Therefore, a large part of the management of JHS involves improving the function and strength of hypermobile joints in order to prevent further problems.

MANAGEMENT OF MUSCULOSKELETAL SYMPTOMS

Acute injuries

Hypermobile individuals can be expected to suffer similar musculoskeletal complaints to non-hypermobile people, although there is evidence to suggest that the risk of developing such complaints is increased in JHS (Hudson et al. 1998, Acasuso-Diaz et al. 1993). Many JHS patients present with an acute injury or acute symptoms at several sites. This may be on a background of long-standing pain in other areas. El-Shahaly and El-Sherif (1991) found that patients complained of several soft tissue complaints, such as bursitis and tendonitis. Management of these acute injuries or flare-ups should follow the same principles as treatment for non-hypermobile patients. They usually respond well to standard physiotherapy modalities of ice, soft tissue massage, electrotherapy, support and rest, followed by gradual mobilization and a return to normal activities. The only difference with the JHS patient is that they take longer to heal, and there may be an increased risk of deconditioning occurring sooner or to a greater extent (Rose 1985). They also need more in the way of reassurance and education regarding future management. Non-steroidal anti-inflammatory medications (NSAIDs), although often reported by patients as being unhelpful, are worth trying in the acute phase where inflammation is present.

The most important aspect of treatment at this stage is to reduce the stress on the injured tissues.

Splinting and support are very valuable to unload the injured or painful tissues, and often need to be used for longer in the hypermobile patient. Care should be taken to avoid dependency, but it is often appropriate to recommend use of the support after the acute injury has recovered, for certain aggravating or potentially overloading situations which may occur as normal everyday activities are resumed. Tape can be used very effectively to unload and support tissues while re-educating and allowing normal movement. Extra care needs to be taken with regard to the increased potential of the JHS patient for skin fragility and irritation.

Subacute and chronic pain

Once the acute injury has settled, attention needs to focus on restoring normal function. The principles of treatment discussed here are applicable for all three symptom presentations referred to earlier and involve restoring a normal range of movement, that is, a normal range of movement for that patient, even if it is a hypermobile range, and gaining efficient muscular control throughout the entire range.

Restoration of normal joint motion

An acute strain or sprain at a joint often results in secondary joint stiffness as the injury settles. This is partly because the patient is frightened to move because it hurts and is fearful of doing further damage, and also because of protective muscle spasm. If normal joint movement is not restored there is the potential to put strain on other adjacent joints and tissues as the body compensates for the lack of movement. This can lead to movement impairments at other sites and may explain the clinical observation, seen frequently with hypermobile patients, of symptoms arising in another area as the original problem area settles. This concept is illustrated by Sahrmann (2002), who describes the body as made up of a series of springs of different tensions. Movement occurs more readily at an area of relatively less tension

than in an area of increased tension or stiffness. This has the potential to set up a pattern of movement which produces stress at an adjacent hypermobile joint, leading to problems at this site through overuse or misuse.

It is interesting to note that Lewkonia and Ansell (1983) reported that a high hypermobility score does not correlate with increased symptoms. This may be because those with marginal scores who do report more symptoms are doing so because of stiffness from previous injury. Unresolved stiffness after injury may mean the patient has not achieved full resolution of the injury and restoration of their normal movement, which could continue to produce symptoms.

Long-standing stiffness, encountered frequently in the thoracic spine, responds well to passive mobilization techniques. Care needs to be taken to ensure that movement is occurring where it is intended to occur. It can be easy to produce movement (and potentially strain) in a hypermobile lumbar spine while mobilizing a stiff thoracic spine. Positioning and support to the hypermobile area are important in order to prevent this happening. Generally, manipulation in the form of thrust techniques is not recommended in the hypermobile patient, because of the risk of overstretching a hypermobile joint. However, thrust techniques can be applied safely and effectively to a stiff thoracic spine if minimal force is used and particular care is taken to isolate the technique to the hypomobile joint.

During manual therapy, it is important to pay attention to what is happening at the joint being passively mobilized, particularly if the joint restriction is thought to be due to muscle spasm. Clinical experience suggests that slow, rhythmic oscillations are most effective, and that once accessory joint movement has been restored the mobilization should cease. This often occurs quickly, and continued mobilization at this stage will result in considerable treatment soreness or an exacerbation of symptoms.

Despite restoration of passive joint movement, it is easy for the patient to continue to move as when they were injured. Therefore, once passive joint movement has been restored in a particular area, re-education of active movement using the restored range is started. This may involve teaching the patient automobilization techniques to maintain the range, and re-educating muscular control of the restored range.

Proprioception has been shown to be defective in hypermobile joints (Hall et al. 1995, Mallik et al. 1994), and consequently JHS patients frequently have difficulty in effectively isolating movement to a particular area. Exercises to improve joint position sense are an essential part of treatment, and the use of mirrors, biofeedback and tape to increase proprioception of the area is useful.

A stiff thoracic spine is a frequent finding in hypermobile patients complaining of back pain. Extension of the spine often occurs excessively in the lumbar spine, with little or no movement in the thoracic spine. Following mobilization of the thoracic joints to restore mobility, the patient needs to learn a new pattern of movement, which involves producing active extension in the area without producing extension in the more mobile lumbar spine. This can be practised in various positions. Four-point kneeling is useful to encourage the patient to straighten the thoracic spine while maintaining a neutral lumbar spine. This is then progressed to performing thoracic spine extension in sitting and standing with lumbar spine control. Lumbar spine control requires activation of the trunk stability muscles, and this is discussed later in the chapter. It is also helpful to teach the patient automobilization techniques to maintain mobility in the area once it has been restored. This may involve either lying over (or extending over while in a sitting position) a rolled-up towel or a ball, positioned in the stiff area. In both instances it is important to ensure that the patient can control the movement effectively before giving it as an exercise to practise on their own. Tape applied to the thoracic spine in a neutral position can be helpful in the re-education process. It helps to:

- Focus attention on the area through enhanced proprioception (Sharma and Pai 1997);

- Support the area in a better position, relieving lengthened, strained, soft tissues; and to
- Prevent the patient slipping back into poor postural habits.

Another area which is frequently found to be stiff in hypermobile patients is the cervicothoracic junction. This can lead to poor movement patterns which involve overusing the more mobile mid-cervical spine, often producing neck and yoke pain. Mobilization to this area, in conjunction with educating a better movement pattern, helps to resolve the problem and prevent recurrences.

Several of our patients have found automobilization techniques, and even the use of such equipment as the 'backnobber' (Fig. 7.1), helpful in relieving stiffness in these areas.

Stretching

Anecdotally, stretching is often reported by hypermobile patients to be helpful in alleviating pain. This may be because they like moving into the end of their range, which they would not normally do during everyday activities, and also as it may relieve feelings of muscular stiffness. It is possible that hypermobile patients have to work their muscles harder to produce stability, and frequently they are seen to use global muscles

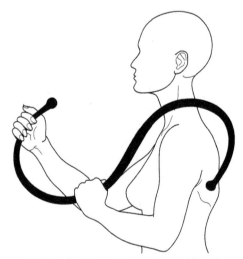

Figure 7.1 'Backnobber' being used to mobilize the upper thoracic spine (Reproduced by permission of The Pressure Positive Company, Gilbertsville, PA, USA.)

rather than postural muscles to achieve this. Sustained contraction of their muscles produces increased tension, ischaemia and fatigue, which can be relieved somewhat by stretching, which improves flexibility and circulation to the muscles. Heat has also been found to be beneficial, particularly prior to stretching. Many hypermobile patients also report being advised not to stretch for fear of damaging their tissues through overstretching. It is potentially easier for a hypermobile person to overstretch, partly as they have increased movement but also as they may lack adequate joint proprioception (Hall et al. 1995). As many patients report benefit from stretching, the important point here is to make sure that the stretch is occurring in an even and controlled way, and that it is happening in the area it is meant to be occurring in. Stretching should be performed in order to maintain the length of muscles and the range of joint movement, rather than increase an already hypermobile range.

Management of movement dysfunction

In order to minimize trauma and the subsequent development of symptoms associated with hypermobile joints, it is essential to prevent and correct movement impairments by improving muscle control throughout the range of movement in hypermobile joints.

Static postures frequently cause problems. Many of us maintain static postures by resting at the end of our joint range. In sitting this leads to a slumped spinal position, and in standing it can lead to locking the knees into extension. These are tempting positions at first, as they are more comfortable than the effort of using muscles to support the joint(s). However, as every physiotherapist knows, these positions mean resting on ligaments and soft tissues at the end of their range. This causes ligament creep and gradual elongation, which can lead to strain and give rise to more pain in the long term. In the hypermobile patient the collagenous tissue is less resilient and more

easily stretched and stressed. This therefore has the potential to weaken and damage the restraining soft tissues around the joint(s) permanently.

It follows therefore that hypermobile patients should be encouraged to maintain a neutral joint position, either actively or passively, when sustaining static postures in order to prevent pain and discomfort. Maintaining a neutral position involves developing a better awareness of body posture in space and better joint position sense. It is potentially more tiring for hypermobile people to maintain a neutral position, as it seems they need to expend more muscle work to control the enlarged neutral zone (Panjabi 1992) and therefore also need to improve the endurance and control of their deep postural muscles to provide additional support to the joint(s). Controlling a hypermobile joint can be difficult and often leads to muscle fatigue, which may contribute to the symptoms of tiredness frequently reported by patients. Hypermobility alone does not necessarily cause pain, but hypermobility with poor control, causing movement dysfunction, can produce stresses which ultimately cause symptoms. It follows, therefore, that treatment should aim to improve the control of hypermobile joints that are causing a movement dysfunction.

Re-education of muscle control often needs to start with improving trunk stability, particularly if the patient has spinal symptoms. Because of the deficit in joint proprioception, it is frequently necessary to teach the patient to find a neutral pelvic position. This is best done in a non-weight-bearing position, such as crook lying, to ensure no symptoms are produced. Once this has been achieved they can progress to activating their trunk stability muscles, starting with transversus abdominis (TrAb). This is often a difficult muscle for patients to 'find'. It may be necessary to try different positions until both physiotherapist and patient are satisfied that they are getting a correct contraction. The use of EMG and pressure biofeedback, mirrors and palpation of the muscle are helpful. Four-point kneeling is an excellent position, but is frequently not possible with hypermobile patients who have knee or wrist problems.

An alternative position is prone lying, which has the added benefit of increased proprioception through contact of the abdomen with the couch.

It is important that the physiotherapist is alert for compensatory strategies that may be employed by the patient. These include activation of the external oblique muscle and breath-holding. Clinical experience has shown that successful activation of the TrAb muscle is often more easily performed by initiating a pelvic floor contraction. Again, the physiotherapist needs to ensure there are no other compensatory movements, such as gluteal and thigh muscle contraction, or movement of the pelvis. It is helpful to include some information on the anatomy of the muscles and the role they play, so the patient has an understanding of why they are being asked to do these exercises.

Once the patient has 'found' the muscle and can produce a contraction, attention should be focused on breathing control. From the outset, patients should be encouraged to activate the TrAb while breathing out, to prevent a common strategy of 'sucking the stomach in'. This is then progressed to maintaining a contraction while breathing normally. Patients frequently have difficulty in breathing with the diaphragm, and it may be necessary to teach lateral costal breathing first and add activation of the TrAb muscle once this has been achieved. Developing effective lateral costal breathing also helps to inhibit activation of the external oblique, where this is over-dominant. Feedback is very useful in the form of feeling where movement is occurring, seeing where movement is occurring by using a mirror, and the use of a towel around the lower ribs to give additional proprioception.

Trunk stability requires these muscles to work in a coordinated way to form a strong cylinder around the lumbar spine to improve control of the neutral zone. The contraction of the muscles should be at a submaximal level – <30–40% of maximum voluntary contraction (Richardson et al. 1999) – and they will need to be trained to work effectively for long periods of time and in different positions. The endurance time is built up slowly, with an emphasis on quality rather than quantity.

Once the patient is confidently able to produce an effective coordinated contraction with minimal effort, the exercise can be progressed to make it more challenging. This involves continuing the training during sitting and standing, which does not require specific time to be set aside for exercising as it can easily be incorporated into everyday life. However, it is also necessary to include exercises that involve maintaining a stable lumbar spine while moving – for example moving a limb – which will challenge the lumbar spine as the centre of gravity is moved. This requires concentration and a well-developed joint position sense in order to appreciate when the lumbar spine is moving. Exercises such as flexing, or abducting the hip while in crook lying, will challenge the lumbar spine by producing a flexion or rotatory movement to the lumbar spine. Feedback can be provided by using a biofeedback bag under the lumbar spine, or using the hands lightly in contact with the pelvis. Another very useful position is four-point kneeling (if this can be tolerated) where the spine is challenged by lifting the leg or arm. This position can also be used in combination with rhythmical stabilizations to improve joint position sense.

Effective trunk stability is necessary for all JHS patients, but those who suffer with back problems may also need additional specific exercises to improve the function of the multifidus muscle. Hides et al. (1994) found that there was a decrease in the size of multifidus, on the side of the pain and at the level of the problem, within 24 hours of the onset of pain. It is not known what this change in size means in terms of muscle function, but there is evidence that improving the function of the multifidus and the other trunk stability muscles is effective in the treatment of low back pain (O'Sullivan 2000, Richardson et al. 1999).

Exercises need to be progressed into weight-bearing and functional positions, particularly those that produce symptoms for the patient. In conjunction with this it is often necessary to spend time improving the patient's posture and postural awareness. JHS patients need to develop an awareness of positioning their joints in a neutral position with even weight-bearing and good alignment, particularly when sustaining static postures. Activation of the trunk stability muscles can be added and exercises progressed to maintaining good posture and stability when their balance is challenged, as in standing or sitting on a balance board, or exercising on a Swiss ball (see Figs 8.2 and 8.4).

Improving spinal stability and postural awareness is frequently the starting point in improving symptoms attributed to hypermobility at the knee and hip. Once this has been achieved, treatment can move on to address the individual problems at these joints.

Hyperextension at the knee is a common finding in the JHS patient and can cause other faults around the knee. The patella tends to be more inferior, possibly owing to decreased activity in the quadriceps muscle (Sahrmann 2002). This can cause irritation of the fat pad and hypermobility or instability of the patella. In addition to advising the patient to stop resting at the end of range of extension, it is necessary to improve control of the last few degrees of extension. This is best achieved using closed chain exercises, with minimal weight-bearing to start with, such as practising knee flexion and extension through a few degrees while the foot is positioned on a Swiss ball. This can be progressed to weight-bearing in standing on both legs, and later on one leg. At all times attention should be given to achieving as correct an alignment as possible throughout the leg, and involves co-contraction of the thigh muscles, pelvis and hip control, and control of overpronation in the feet. A Total Gym (Fig. 7.2) (San Diego, CA) has been found to be particularly useful in the clinic as the amount of weight taken through the limb can be gradually increased. It also facilitates an appreciation of how 'wobbly' the movement often is in hypermobile patients, who have difficulty maintaining the movement in the sagittal plane.

The hip joint is frequently a cause of symptoms in the JHS patient, the most common problems being hyperextension, clicking or subluxation. Prolonged standing in hyperextension produces excessive flexibility in the anterior hip structures and can lead to femoral anterior glide syndrome (Sahrmann 2002). This is thought to cause pain through overstretching of anterior hip structures and pinching of the anterior hip capsule in flexion. It is frequently seen in combination with weak long iliopsoas muscles, weak hip extensors and dominant, stronger tensor fascia lata (TFL) and hamstrings. The dominance of TFL in comparison to posterior gluteus medius produces hip medial rotation, seen in walking and one-leg stance. Treatment to correct this movement fault involves educating the patient to avoid unhelpful postures, such as sitting in a 'W' (Fig. 7.3), which increases hip medial rotation and standing in a sway posture. They should be taught to maintain

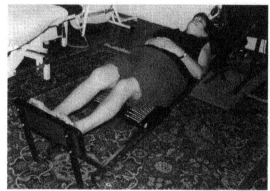

Figure 7.2 Improving stability around the knee using the Total Gym

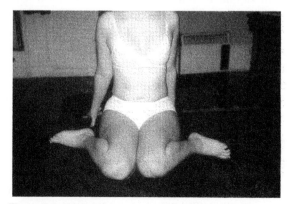

Figure 7.3 Unhelpful postures. Sitting in a 'W' position

correct alignment in standing and walking, and given exercises to increase the strength of the hip flexors and gluteal muscles, particularly posterior gluteus medius, to counter hip medial rotation. Patients can be taught to contract their gluteal muscles during heel strike and on moving from sitting to standing, so that it becomes a part of everyday life.

The management of problems commonly associated with the neck and shoulder joints and the feet in hypermobile patients are discussed in detail in Chapter 5.

JHS patients frequently report symptoms associated with the temporomandibular joint (TMJ) and usually present in one of two ways. Pain in the area of the joint is reported in association with stiffness and reduced jaw opening due to muscle spasm; or at the other end of the scale patients report a feeling of 'looseness' in the joint, with clicking, subluxation or dislocation on wide opening of the jaw.

Treatment is guided by examination findings, but in the case of the stiff TMJ normal movement can be restored through joint mobilization and muscle relaxation techniques applied to the muscles around the jaw, in particular the masseter. Treatment of the lax TMJ is aimed at reducing the occurrence of subluxation by avoiding wide jaw opening, as in eating an apple or French bread. Stability can be improved by rhythmic stabilizations applied to the mandible. The upper cervical spine is frequently associated with TMJ dysfunction. Mobilization to this area, in combination with exercises to improve the stabilizing function of the deep neck flexor muscles (Jull 1997) and attention to head on neck posture, is important (Bryden and Fitzgerald 2001). Readers are directed to the book by Kraus (1994) for further detail on the management of TMJ dysfunction.

Management of symptoms associated with pregnancy

Although it is thought that increased mobility in the sacroiliac (SI) joints in response to hormones is responsible for peripartum pelvic pain (PPPP), it is not known whether hypermobile women are more at risk. However, clinical experience suggests that many hypermobile women do have problems associated with their SI joints during pregnancy.

It is not possible to measure accurately the mobility of the SI joints, but it is possible that it is the difference in mobility between the two SI joints that is important in the production of pain (Pool-Goudzwaard et al. 1998). This is similar to other areas of the body in which relative hypomobility produces increased stress on the hypermobile side. Treatment should be directed at the hypomobile joint to restore mobility. Gentle techniques designed to nutate the sacrum and posteriorly rotate the ilium can be effective in relieving pain and restoring mobility to the hypomobile joint. Patients can be taught to use the transverse abdominal muscles, pelvic floor and gluteal muscles to compensate for instability of the pelvis by increasing the muscle force, but this only works for a short time (Vleeming et al. 1995). Often external support is necessary to provide some stability. A non-elastic pelvic belt, which significantly increases force closure, was found to relieve PPPP in about 50% of women while pregnant and in about two-thirds of women after delivery (Mens et al. 1996). Severe cases of sacroiliac joint instability may need the help of crutches.

Educating the patient about the condition is important so that they can change their lifestyle where possible to accommodate the insufficiency of the pelvis. Activities that stress the pelvis should be avoided, such as climbing stairs, one-leg standing, stepping up on to a high step, such as on to a bus, and extreme movements of the spine or hips. It is thought that the action of iliopsoas leads to a large asymmetric force being placed on the SI joint, which can exacerbate symptoms (Pool-Goudzwaard et al. 1998). Ignoring the pain will not help and will most likely cause an increase in the pain, which is often not felt until the following day (Ostgaard 1998). Rest is recommended, but complete bed rest should be avoided because of its deleterious effect on muscle strength and endurance.

Posterior pelvic pain disappears in the majority of women within 3 months after delivery (Ostgaard 1998). Once the posterior pelvic pain provocation test is negative, showing that the pelvis has regained its stability, specific training of the pelvic floor, back and abdominal muscles should be started. Rehabilitation is slow – between 6 and 12 months – and normally contains periods of relapse (Ostgaard 1998), probably the result of the extra physical work involved in looking after a new baby. Ostgaard (1998) also emphasizes that strenuous work should be avoided for 6 months after delivery even if the pain has disappeared, in order to avoid a relapse later.

Hypermobile patients are invariably concerned about other factors, such as looking after the child, breastfeeding, whether the child will have problems, and the effect of another pregnancy. If they attend the physiotherapist during the pregnancy they may also be concerned about the labour. Generally, caesarean operations are not recommended in cases of low back pain or PPPP (Ostgaard 1998), although caesareans have been recommended in the case of hypermobility type III Ehlers–Danlos syndrome (Charvet et al. 1991). Advice to help during the labour is useful, and sometimes speaking to the consultant or midwife can relieve some of the patient's anxiety. It is not known which is the best position for delivery, but it would seem advisable to support the patient's legs and back and prevent excessive unsupported hip abduction.

EDUCATION AND ADVICE

Patients who have been suffering from pain for a long time and who have not been recognized as being hypermobile feel a huge sense of relief when a diagnosis and an explanation for their problems is finally given. Reassurance that they are not suffering from a progressive rheumatological complaint and that there is a reason for their symptoms reduces anxiety and allows them to focus on ways of managing the problem.

Education about the condition forms one of the most important aspects of treatment given by a physiotherapist, and understanding the implications of the disorder may help them to cope with their pain more effectively (Russek 1999).

It is important to give patients a clear understanding of how to look after their joints without causing undue concern or worry. They should not be fearful of using their joints, but rather made aware of activities or situations that make their joints and tissues more vulnerable to injury.

The initial assessment of a patient will give the physiotherapist an indication of particular areas where potential problems may develop and allow them to give specific advice to the patient. This often involves questioning the patient in detail about their daily activities. Advice generally concerns two aspects: avoidance of potentially harmful postures, usually involving maintaining joints at end of range, and reducing the time spent in repetitive activities.

Sustaining harmful postures

In standing, patients should avoid sustaining hyperextension at the knee, which is thought to contribute to patellofemoral joint problems (Al-Rawi and Nessan 1997), 'hanging' on one hip or standing in a sway posture, and sustaining hyperextension of the hips. Buttressing the knees together while standing, or on moving from sitting to standing, is a habit which affects hypermobile and non-hypermobile subjects alike and can lead to a strain of the medial compartment of the knee. Patients should also be advised to avoid sitting with the legs outstretched and the knees unsupported, sitting in a 'W', sitting with the leg tucked under the buttock, or sitting cross-legged 'Indian style'. These positions have the potential to stretch the collateral ligaments of the knee (Shoen et al. 1982). Prolonged kneeling with the weight taken on the ankles in full plantar flexion was responsible for a severe strain of the ankle and anterior tibial muscles in a patient in our clinic. Another patient reported a 7-year history of thoracic spine pain after sitting on the floor with the legs outstretched and the thoracic spine rotated to the left for a few hours. Many hypermobile patients like to rest on the lateral border of their feet in standing or sitting, producing a sustained stretch to the lateral ankle. While sleeping they should avoid sustained rotation of the head, as in lying prone, and sustained wrist and elbow flexion, which was found to be responsible for carpal tunnel symptoms (March et al. 1988).

Repetitive activities

Repetitive activities cannot be avoided at work or at home, but the patient should be advised to perform them as symmetrically as possible and not to prolong them for too long. There is no answer to the question 'how long is too long?' It will depend on the patient, the activity and the situation. Details of the activities regularly performed by the patient can be analysed and suggestions made to reduce the stress on joints and tissues. As a general guide, if a particular activity is producing pain, the maximum time the activity can be performed without symptoms should be noted and reduced to 75% initially, and then increased gradually as the symptoms subside.

Activities around the home which have been given as reasons for the onset of pain or an increase in existing pain by our patients are decorating, DIY, gardening, digging or pruning, cooking, a lot of chopping or beating, as in making a cake, activities performed with the arms above shoulder height, and vacuuming. There are many tips that the physiotherapist can give to the hypermobile patient to help them improve their activities around the house and garden. Taking regular breaks and varying activities as much as possible during the day is helpful. Much of the advice given to people with back pain can be applied to good effect. Ensuring that work surfaces around the home are at the correct height when performing lengthy tasks will help to avoid strain. The use of

a separate wheeled trolley at the correct height can make up for surfaces that are not at an ideal height in the kitchen. Likewise, using another bowl turned upside down in the sink, or a bowl on the draining board, can help washing-up to be achieved at a comfortable height. Hand-washing clothes can be done with less pain and effort by using nailbrushes with handles. It is also worth investigating whether there are any aids available, such as garden equipment designed for arthritic hands. In order to continue doing some activities which either have to be done or are done for enjoyment, it may be prudent to advise the patient on suitable supports to be used while performing the activity.

Housework can be thought of as exercise and it can be a good opportunity for patients to practise and put into use exercises that help trunk stability. Developing efficient trunk stability while being active will reduce the tendency for household activities, particularly those that involve bending or sustained postures, to produce symptoms.

Work postures and activities frequently cause problems in hypermobile patients. Work-related dysfunction can be prevented and helped by regular rest periods, in combination with gentle mobilizing and stretching exercises, attention to good posture and symmetrical working practices. It may be necessary to arrange an on-site assessment to fully appreciate and advise on improving working conditions. At its worst, if unmanageable symptoms persist a career change may have to be considered. More information on work-related problems is given in Chapter 9.

LIFESTYLE MODIFICATIONS

Sleeping

JHS patients often awake with pain and stiffness. This may be due partly to the mattress being too hard. Many patients buy an orthopaedic or harder mattress in the belief that it will help their back pain. This is frequently not the case, and hypermobile people are often more comfortable with a softer mattress. This problem can be helped by overlaying the mattress with a duvet or piece of foam as a temporary measure. If a trial of this appears to help their morning symptoms and improves their night's sleep, then a more permanent overlay mattress can be purchased. A pocket-sprung mattress, although expensive, is often the best, although the beneficial effect of this can be cancelled out by a hard, unsprung base. Try to find a manufacturer that will allow the bed to be returned if it proves unsatisfactory.

Sharing the bed with a heavy partner may be a problem by causing the mattress to dip into the middle. This can be helped somewhat by an overlay mattress on the side of the lighter person. A better resolution to the problem is to buy a mattress that is made up of two single mattresses, each made to the individual person's specifications.

Feather pillows are less 'springy' than foam ones and are often more comfortable for hypermobile patients with neck problems. They can be shaped to individual requirements and, if necessary, some of the feathers can be removed to make moulding the pillow easier. A good alternative to feathers is pressure-sensitive foam, which has been on the market more recently. It was designed for the space programme and is made with high-density foam that responds to heat and pressure by softening and moulding itself around the object it is supporting. On release of the pressure it returns to its original shape.

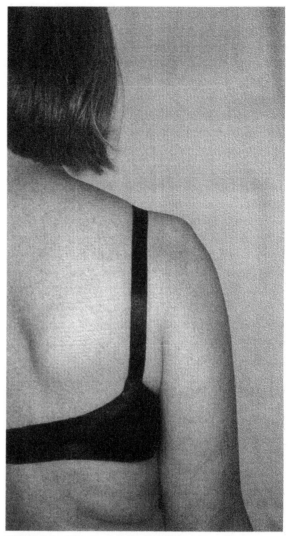

Figure 7.4 Effect on a hypermobile shoulder of carrying a light load

Carrying

Some activities may put certain joints under particular stress. Shoulders that are potentially unstable, particularly in an inferior direction, can be put under stress with relatively light carrying. Figure 7.4 shows the effect on a hypermobile shoulder of carrying a carrier bag in the hand. The shoulder is clearly under stress, with the weight of the bag in the dependent hand producing an inferior subluxation, even under light loading. There is obviously a case for specific exercises to improve the stability of the shoulder in this case, including attention to strength and endurance. However, it is unlikely that a shoulder with this degree of hypermobility will be able to sustain heavy loads, or even light carrying, for a prolonged period.

Commonsense advice can be helpful. It is better to shop for smaller quantities more frequently and to distribute the load evenly between both sides. Wearing gloves when carrying plastic bags can provide a cushioning effect to the hands.

Shopping trolleys are not just for the elderly and can make a huge difference to shopping for the family. In the supermarket it is less stressful to the joints to use the smaller lighter trolleys, if possible. It is easier for the shorter person to turn the trolley through 90° and push through the long side. The ideal way to avoid carrying heavy loads is to have a lot of the heavier staple items of shopping delivered to the door. Handbags and briefcases should be as light as possible, and depending on the problem areas it may be better for a patient to use a rucksack or 'bumbag'.

Changes to lifestyle have to be considered and patients may have to make difficult decisions that affect not only themselves but also their families. Giving patients an understanding of how a simple everyday activity can affect their joints will help them to understand how they can prevent and control the amount of stress they subject their joints to in the future.

Clothing

Clothing is best if it is light and not too tight. A surprisingly small amount of pressure seems to trigger muscle tension, especially in patients with spinal problems. For women with large breasts a well-fitting bra with wider straps and a crossover at the back can help to reduce yoke pain and improve thoracic posture at the same time. Unfortunately, some women find that crossover straps trigger a stiffening of the thoracic spine. As with most things, the only way to find out, is through trial and error.

Footwear

Shoes can also cause problems by provoking painful feet. Soft, light, supportive shoes with flexible soles appear to be best. Because of the tendency towards increased fragility of the skin (Mishra et al. 1996), high stiff backs in shoes should be avoided as they can precipitate Achilles tendonitis. It is worth knowing that it is often possible to undo the stitching at the back of training shoes and take out some of the rigid material. Shock-absorbing insoles or even heel pads can help, although custom-made orthotics may be necessary to provide adequate support for the feet.

Travelling

Travelling on holiday can involve many anxieties for the JHS patient. Packing for the family is best started early, long before departure. Trains are easier to cope with than planes, as there is more room to move around. If flying, the patient should be encouraged to exercise regularly during the flight. Small mobility and stretching exercises can be done for most joints, and a regular walk up and down the cabin every 1–2 hours will help to prevent stiffness and tiredness. If this is not enough then a short jog on the spot for 2–3 minutes may help (for privacy use the washroom). Most airlines will allow a person to take any equipment necessary for their medical condition as extra luggage if packed in a separate bag. It may be helpful for a hypermobile patient to take cushions, pillows or supports to make the journey more comfortable. A letter from the doctor or physiotherapist may be required. If it is possible to upgrade to business class the journey and recovery period will be much easier.

While on holiday a blow-up mattress can transform the beach or sunbed into a relaxing place. A piece of foam can be taken in the luggage to improve an unfamiliar bed, and even better, but more expensive, is a compact, self-inflating sleeping mattress that can be found in camping shops.

While travelling, a supportive chair may not be available, and at these times cushions or pieces of foam, or even a rolled-up coat, can help to make the person more comfortable and well supported. A cushion can be hidden inside a plastic bag or a soft handbag so that carrying it need not cause embarrassment. There is no need to take it out of its cover, as the whole thing can be used as a cushion. Blow-up cushions are especially useful when travelling, for use behind the neck, behind the back, to sit on, or even under the feet if the chair is too high.

Hypermobile patients usually like to be supported by cushions: the softer the support the better. They are generally uncomfortable people, and finding the right chair, bed, pillows, shoes etc. is very important to them. They are often very fussy, but for a good reason, and the right equipment will make a tremendous difference to their lives.

Family and children

Living with a person who has JHS and who is not in control of their symptoms can be stressful for family and friends. It is often helpful for the physiotherapist to talk to family members and involve them in some of the discussions regarding the condition, the problems being encountered, and how to manage them. Encourage the patient to talk to their family about how they are feeling, and discuss how they can best help them.

Usually family members want to do too much to help, and it is difficult to achieve the right balance between doing too much and doing too little. It is important to keep communicating on what is and is not helpful, and to tell people when they have been helpful. There may be some simple physiotherapy techniques that a family member can be taught to help alleviate pain.

A more complex problem a patient may have to deal with is when they realize that one of their children may be complaining of symptoms of JHS. Apart from dealing with their own pain they have to help the child sort out their anxieties about whether they will develop their parent's problem. If they show symptoms it is necessary to talk to them about the syndrome and reassure them that it may not necessarily mean a poor prognosis. Helping the parent to organize practical solutions for the child and encourage them to give lots of love and sympathy can be beneficial. At some point it may be advisable to have the problem assessed and diagnosed by a rheumatologist. If the diagnosis is confirmed this may be a good time to consult a physiotherapist with regard to general advice on joint care, exercise and fitness, and anything else that is particularly worrying the child. This may also be an appropriate time to consider seeking advice on career choices.

In addition, it is worth bearing in mind that the parent may be dealing with feelings of guilt about passing on this problem to their child.

Having children can make extra physical demands and can worsen the patient's symptoms for quite a long time, especially if they have more than one child. In this case, a gap of about 2½ years between children is more manageable. A mother may have to accept that she needs extra help with the children. If this is possible, a 'mother's help', rather than a nanny, is best, as they can do the heavy work such as shopping, ironing and cleaning.

The symptoms of JHS can change or even first appear during pregnancy. Occasionally women feel much better while pregnant, only for their symptoms to return soon after the birth. In the postnatal period the patient is often tired, and adequate rest and joint positioning during this period is essential. Pleasurable as breastfeeding is for both mother and baby, the positioning can provoke a great deal of spinal pain. One welltried technique is to sit in a wide armchair or bed with the back supported. Place two pillows in an inverted 'V', overlapping at the point of the lap. The baby's legs can then be placed under the mother's arm so that the head is resting near the adjacent breast. The mother can then relax back and feed and talk to the baby at the same time, without having to use her arms to support the baby. Everything to do with a newborn baby or small child involves bending. Increasing the height of much-used items such as the changing table and cot will reduce the bending as much as possible.

Other health issues

There may be other areas of the JHS patient's life that are worrying them and with which the physiotherapist can help.

Visits to the dentist can be difficult, and it may be necessary to discuss how the condition affects the patient with the dentist before treatment is started. The patient's treatment may mean more visits than for other people, as it is often difficult for the dentist to differentiate a dental pain from musculoskeletal pain being referred from the neck or TMJ. The physiotherapist should be able to help with the differential diagnosis.

The dentist may have limited access to the mouth because of restricted opening due to stiffness in the TMJ. Prolonged work in the mouth can cause increased pain for the patient, either in the TMJ or in the upper cervical spine. Patients should be warned to advise their dentist about the problem and ensure that the mouth is not held open for too long or with too much vigour. A prop is not recommended as it holds the jaw in a stretched position with no control from the patient. The position of the neck is also important. Modern dental chairs can convert into a flat couch on which the patient can lie with their neck supported by a cushion. A flat mattress, such as from a garden chair, overlaying the couch will give support to the back and shoulders if this is necessary. Not all dentists are aware that local anaesthetic injections are less effective in many JHS patients than in other people.

A JHS patient will recover more quickly after a major operation if they remain in hospital a little longer than usual. It is also vital to inform the surgeon, obstetrician or anaesthetist about the condition, so that extra care can be taken of the head and neck by the theatre staff when moving the patient during the operation. It may be advisable for the patient to wear a collar, to provide support and remind staff that extra care is needed.

Management of related symptoms

There may be several other medical problems that the patient has not mentioned to the physiotherapist, as they do not associate them with their hypermobility. These can result from the involvement of other body systems owing to the patient's collagen defect. It can be a great relief to the patient to realize that there is one reason for their many complaints.

Varicose veins can lead to venous insufficiency, causing tired and aching legs. Support stockings can help, as does a reduction in excess weight.

The skin can bruise and blister more easily because of the increased fragility of the skin and blood vessels (El-Garf et al. 1998, Al-Rawi et al. 1985, Grahame et al. 1981, Mishra et al. 1996). Special gel plasters can act as an effective prophylaxis, and a second skin dressing promotes healing.

Urogenital dysfunction, including stress incontinence, may be helped by specialist physiotherapy, although if it is more than mild, assessment by a urogenital surgeon may be appropriate. Because of the proximity of the rectum to other organs, constipation may make these symptoms worse. Constipation appears to be common in JHS patients and may be due in part to the use of painkilling drugs. It is important, therefore, that when they start taking painkillers they also take something that produces a soft bulkier stool. Isogel, a natural fibre drink, has this action because it is not absorbed by the gastrointestinal tract, and therefore retains a lot of water.

Patients may report symptoms of hyperventilation, such as chest pain, dizzy spells and paraesthesiae of the lips (personal observation). This may be helped by breathing exercises in the first instance, although referral to a physiotherapist experienced in hyperventilation may be necessary. Some of these symptoms may be due to autonomic neuropathy (see Chapter 1).

Medication

Patients frequently ask questions about medication, either about the medication they are on or if there are any alternatives. Currently physiotherapists cannot prescribe, and any advice and suggestions they make should be discussed with the patient's GP. There follow some suggestions regarding medication that have been found through clinical experience to be helpful to the JHS patient (see Chapter 3).

Valium can be useful for treating increased muscle tension that is causing pain. A small dose is often sufficient and should be used in the short term only. Valium is an antispasmodic drug that works centrally on the CNS and so produces generalized hypotonia. That would be a disadvantage to the JHS patient in the long term; it may also be habit-forming and so long-term use should be avoided.

In the acute phase of an injury non-steroidal anti-inflammatory drugs (NSAIDs) can be helpful, but are best to be avoided in anyone with related gastrointestinal problems. In cases of severe chronic pain a low dose (5–10 mg) daily of amitriptyline can reduce pain and promote better-quality sleep, often so needed in these patients.

Sport and exercise

Although it is important to increase strength and endurance in muscles around the joints and enable patients to be independent of the physiotherapist by encouraging a habit of lifelong exercise, it is not enough to leave the patient to their own devices or the personal trainer at the local gym. Individual advice is very important that takes into account the individual patient's weak areas and movement patterns.

Swimming is frequently suggested as good exercise for hypermobile patients, as it reduces the stresses on the joints while allowing the patient to improve their cardiovascular health. However, it is not enough to just tell a patient to go swimming. Patients with hypermobile shoulders may risk overstretching their shoulder joints through repetitive forceful movements at end of range, in both breaststroke and crawl. An awareness of the problem and a modification of the stroke can reduce this risk. Advice also needs to be given to patients who do not swim with their head in the water, as they risk straining the midcervical joints by prolonged cervical extension. Useful recommendations to improve the posture and reduce

stress on tissues while swimming are contained in the book *The Art of Swimming* by Shaw and D'Angour, based on the Alexander Technique.

Yoga and Pilates are examples of suitable exercise regimens that patients can follow once they have a clear understanding of their vulnerable areas. The topic of general fitness and sport is dealt with in more detail in Chapter 8.

HYPERMOBILITY AND THE PHYSIOTHERAPIST

Physiotherapists, while giving advice to hypermobile patients, need also to consider their own work practices if they are themselves hypermobile. Repeated and prolonged bending over the treatment couch, without active muscle work in the abdominals and glutei, may weaken a hypermobile lumbar spine causing serious consequences for the physiotherapist's future career. Knees can also suffer if held in the hyperextended position or buttressed together while working on a patient. Hypermobility in the thumbs and fingers can be a cause of pain when performing mobilizations (Fig. 7.5) and may necessitate the use of custom-made splints for support to prevent further damage. It is also important that physiotherapists recognize when they or their colleagues are hypermobile so that potentially damaging techniques are not performed on them repeatedly as students.

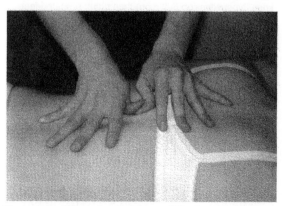

Figure 7.5 Effect of performing mobilization techniques with hypermobile thumbs

Case study

A 21-year-old female student reported suffering knee pain from the age of 7, and throughout her years at school had been aware of pain in her legs during games. This had been largely ignored by the teachers, and repeated visits to the GP were of little help. She felt she was not being listened to and dismissed. She started ice-skating, which helped her flat feet and improved her knee symptoms slightly.

At the age of 12 she fell down stairs and developed pain in her coccyx and low back. Her hands and wrists began hurting during her 'A' levels, and she found they seized up after writing for an hour. She suffered bouts of depression during her teens and was treated with antidepressants. Interestingly, she also reported an unpleasant experience of having four teeth taken out at the age of 10, when the anaesthetic proved ineffective.

During her first year at university she suffered further depression and increased pain in many joints. Her hip joints started to hurt and feel unstable, her shoulders felt as if they would 'come out', particularly with carrying. She was finally investigated by a rheumatologist. All rheumatological tests were negative and she was diagnosed as suffering from JHS.

At the time of the physiotherapy assessment she described her hips and knees as most problematic, but she also had daily pain in her back, knees hands and wrists (Fig. 7.6). The pain varied from 3 to 9 on a scale of 0–10. She described having good and bad days: a good day was a day when nothing hurt and occurred 'practically never'; a bad day was when she was unable to go to college, and these occurred once every 2–3 weeks. She was unable to walk to college once a week. It was seriously affecting her social life, as she was frequently unable to go out at night and unable to dance. Her main aim from treatment was 'to get through a day without joint pain'.

Her general health was good, although she suffered bouts of fatigue for a day every 2 weeks for no apparent reason. Anti-inflammatory medication was no help. Sleep was unaffected, but she often woke feeling achy and stiff, and felt tired by the end of the day, finding it 'an effort to stay upright'.

On examination she was found to stand with a kyphosis–lordosis posture in anterior pelvic tilt, with slight knee hyperextension (left more than right), pronated feet (although she had learnt to control this somewhat), forward head posture and increased tension in the upper trapezius muscles. In walking there was an increase in lumbar extension and poor stability around the pelvis when standing on one leg.

Spinal flexion was surprisingly limited to the mid shin and produced pain in the hips and demonstrated increased flexion in the thoracic spine, a flat lumbar spine and tightness of the hips and hamstrings. Hip pain was increased and pain produced in the calves with the addition of neck flexion. Spinal extension was excessive and produced solely in the lumbar spine. Lateral flexion was asymmetrical, with the fingertips reaching to 2 in. below the knee crease to the left and 4 in. on the right. She showed widespread hypermobility in her joints, scoring 6/9 on the Beighton scale and 7/9 historically. Outside of the scale her patellae, shoulders, cervical spine and finger joints were also hypermobile. The hip joints showed increased medial rotation and adduction (left more than right), with pain at the end of range. Flexion was also restricted and produced anterior groin pain. Straight leg raise (SLR) was restricted by tension in the hamstrings, pain in the calf and hip at 60° on the right and 70° on the left. Further tests demonstrated muscle imbalance around the hip, with dominant hamstrings, weak gluteal muscles and tight calf muscles.

At the end of the examination the findings were discussed with the patient and a treatment plan agreed. The main elements of this were to improve neural mobility and thoracic mobility into extension, combined with an exercise programme to increase the stiffness and control of the lumbar spine, particularly into extension, and improve recruitment and strength of the hip extensors and lateral rotators. She was given instruction in 'finding' a neutral pelvic position in crook lying and started on activating TrAb though a pelvic floor contraction with good breathing control.

Subsequent treatment sessions included manual therapy to the thoracic spine and neural mobilization in combination with soft tissue techniques, including hold/relax to improve flexibility in the calf and hamstring muscles. She responded relatively quickly and achieved her normal range of spinal flexion, being able to place her fingertips on the floor with a more even spinal curve and no pain after three sessions. SLR with dorsiflexion likewise improved to 80° each side, with only slight hamstring tension. In addition, trunk stability work was progressed, with time spent on improving posture and encouraging the use of abdominal and gluteal muscles when moving from sitting to standing, standing and walking. Particular attention was paid to re-educating the use of gluteus maximus to produce hip extension, with lumbar spine control and strengthening posterior gluteus medius. Later, exercises were included to improve the stability and control of hyperextension at the knees.

As frequently seems to happen with hypermobile patients, once one area is under control another causes a problem. This patient had a recurrence of pain in her elbows, neck and right shoulder, and her fingers had seized up during a period of writing in an examination. However, she felt more in control of these symptoms and they were less severe than previously, primarily because she felt able to control them through attention to posture, performing gentle stretching exercises and taking regular breaks. She was given additional advice and specific exercises to improve stability and control of the shoulder girdle, through improved function of the lower trapezius and deep neck flexor muscle training.

After 10 sessions over a 4-month period she reported feeling more positive and more in control. She had not had any really bad days and was experiencing several days with no pain at all. Her hips felt more stable, 'not even threatening to come out', and she had managed to do an active sightseeing trip around a city feeling only tired rather than in pain. She rated her pain as 0/10 at its best and 5/10 at its worst. The worst times were, however, short-lived and often associated with sitting in 'bizarre positions'.

Time was also spent educating the patient on JHS and answering particular concerns. Some of these were regarding her career and how she would cope with having children.

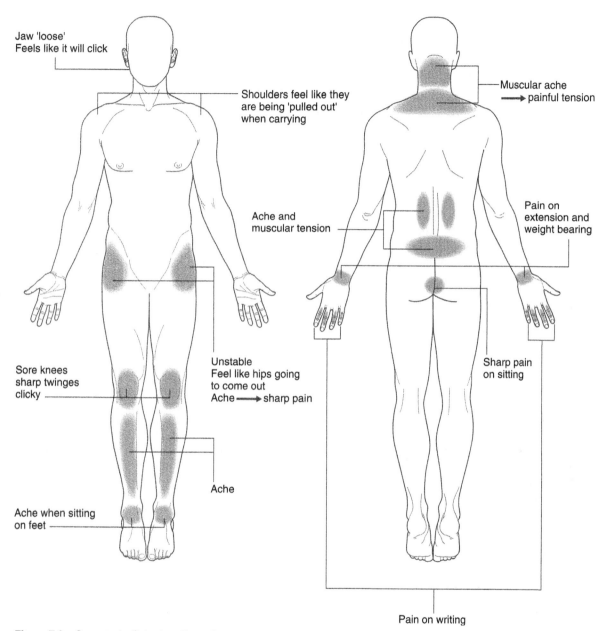

Jaw 'loose'
Feels like it will click

Shoulders feel like they
are being 'pulled out'
when carrying

Muscular ache
⟶ painful tension

Ache and
muscular tension

Pain on
extension and
weight bearing

Sore knees
sharp twinges
clicky

Unstable
Feel like hips going
to come out
Ache ⟶ sharp pain

Sharp pain
on sitting

Ache

Ache when sitting
on feet

Pain on writing

Figure 7.6   Case study: Pain chart illustrating symptoms at time of assessment

CONCLUSION

For many, hypermobility does not cause a problem and can even be seen as an asset. For others, less fortunate, their hypermobility brings with it numerous, widespread and long-standing musculoskeletal symptoms, which may have been mismanaged in the past. This presents a challenge for the physiotherapist, but it is one that is often rewarding. Treatment involves the use of many skills, including mobilization, exercise to improve posture, muscle balance and endurance, proprioception and joint awareness. It also involves reassurance, education and, where necessary, some lifestyle modifications to enable the patient to manage the condition more effectively and independently.

REFERENCES

Acasuso-Diaz, M., Collantes-Estevez, E. and Sánchez Guijo, P. (1993) Joint hyperlaxity and musculoligamentous lesions: study of a population of homogeneous age, sex and physical exertion. *British Journal of Rheumatology*, **32**, 120–2.

Al-Rawi, Z.S., Al-Aszawi, A.J. and Al-Chalabi, T. (1985) Joint mobility among university students in Iraq. *British Journal of Rheumatology*, **4**, 326–31.

Al-Rawi, Z. and Nessan, A.H. (1997) Joint hypermobility in patients with chondromalacia patellae. *British Journal of Rheumatology*, **12**, 1324–7.

Bryden, L. and Fitzgerald, D. (2001) The influence of posture and alteration of function. In: *Craniofacial Dysfunction and Pain: Manual Therapy Assessment and Management* (H. von Piekartz and L. Bryden, eds). Butterworth–Heinemann.

Charvet, P.Y., Salle, B., Rebaud, P. et al. (1991) Ehlers–Danlos syndrome and pregnancy. Apropos of a case. (abstract) *Journal of Gynecology Obstetrics Biology and Reproduction* (Paris), **20**, 75–8.

Cherpel, A. and Marks, R. (1999) The benign joint hypermobility syndrome. *New Zealand Journal of Physiotherapy*, **27**, 9–22.

El-Garf, A.K., Mahmoud, G.A. and Mahgoub, E.H. (1998) Hypermobility among Egyptian children: prevalence and features. *Journal of Rheumatology*, **5**, 1003–5.

El-Shahaly, H.A. and El-Sherif, A.K. (1991) Is the benign hypermobility syndrome benign? *Clinical Rheumatology*, **10**, 302–7.

Finsterbush, A. and Pogrund, H. (1982) The hypermobility syndrome. Musculoskeletal complaints in 100 consecutive cases of generalized joint hypermobility. *Clinical Orthopedics*, **168**, 124–7.

Grahame, R., Edwards, J.C., Pitcher, D. et al. (1981) A clinical and echocardiographic study of patients with the hypermobility syndrome. *Annals of the Rheumatic Diseases*, **40**, 541–6.

Hall, M.G., Ferrell, W.R., Sturrock, R.D. et al. (1995) The effect of the hypermobility syndrome on knee joint proprioception. *British Journal of Rheumatology*, **34**, 121–5.

Hides, J.A., Stokes, M.J., Saide, M. et al. (1994) Evidence of lumbar multifidus muscle wasting ipsilateral to symptoms in patients with acute/subacute low back pain. *Spine*, **19**, 165–72.

Hudson, N., Fitzcharles, M.-A., Cohen, M. et al. (1998) The association of soft tissue rheumatism and hypermobility. *British Journal of Rheumatology*, **37**, 382–6.

Jull, G. (1997) The management of cervicogenic headache. *Manual Therapy*, **2**, 182–90.

Kraus, S.L. (1994) *TMJ Disorders*, 2nd edn. *Clinics in Physical Therapy*. Churchill Livingstone.

Lewkonia, R.M. and Ansell, B.M. (1983) Articular hypermobility simulating chronic rheumatic disease. *Archives of Disease in Childhood*, **58**, 988–92.

Mallik, A.K., Ferrell, W.R., McDonald, A.G. and Sturrock, R.D. (1994) Impaired proprioceptive acuity at the proximal interphalangeal joint in patients with the hypermobility syndrome. *British Journal of Rheumatology*, **33**, 631–7.

March, L.M., Francis, H. and Webb, J. (1988) Benign joint hypermobility with neuropathies: documentation of median, sciatic and common peroneal nerve compression. *Clinical Rheumatology*, **7**, 35–40.

Mens, J.M.A., Vleeming, A., Stoeckart, R. et al. (1996) Understanding peripartum pelvic pain. *Spine*, **21**, 1363–70.

Mishra, M.B., Ryan, P., Atkinson, P. et al. (1996) Extra-articular features of benign joint hypermobility syndrome. *British Journal of Rheumatology*, **35**, 861–6.

O'Sullivan, P.B. (2000) Lumbar segmental 'instability': clinical presentation and specific stabilizing exercise management. *Manual Therapy*, **5**, 2–12.

Ostgaard, H.C. (1998) Assessment and treatment of low back pain in working pregnant women. In: Conference Proceedings Third Interdisciplinary World Congress on Low Back Pain and Pelvic Pain (A. Vleeming et al. eds), pp. 161–171. European Conference Organizers Rotterdam.

Panjabi, M.M. (1992) The stabilizing system of the spine. Part II. Neutral zone and instability hypothesis. *Journal of Spinal Disorders*, **5**, 390–7.

Pool-Goudzwaard, A.L., Vleeming, A., Stoeckart, R. et al. (1998) Insufficient lumbo-pelvic stability: a clinical, anatomical and biomechanical approach to 'aspecific' low back pain. *Manual Therapy*, **3**, 12–20.

Richardson, C., Jull, G., Hodges, P. and Hides, J. (1999) *Therapeutic Exercise for Spinal Stabilization in Low Back Pain*, p 94. Churchill Livingstone.

Rose, B.S. (1985) The hypermobility syndrome. Loose-limbed and liable. *New Zealand Journal of Physiotherapy*, **13**, 18–19.

Russek, L.N. (1999) Hypermobility syndrome. *Physical Therapy*, **79**, 591–9.

Russek, L.N. (2000) Examination and treatment of a patient with hypermobility syndrome. *Physical Therapy*, **80**, 386–98.

Sahrmann, S. (2002) *Diagnosis and Treatment of Movement Impairment Syndromes*. Mosby.

Sharma, L. and Pai, Y.C. (1997) Impaired proprioception and osteoarthritis. *Current Opinion in Rheumatology*, **3**, 253–8.

Shaw, S. and D'Angour, A. (1996) *The Art of Swimming in a New Direction with the Alexander Technique*. Bath: Ashgrove Publishing.

Shoen, R.P., Kirsner, A.B., Farber, S.J. and Finkel, R.I. (1982) The hypermobility syndrome. *Postgraduate Medicine*, **71**, 199–208.

Vleeming, A., Pool-Goudzwaard, A.L. and Stoeckart, R. (1995) The posterior layer of the thoracolumbar fascia. Its function in load transfer from spine to legs. *Spine*, **20**, 753–8.

8

Rehabilitation, fitness, sport and performance for individuals with joint hypermobility

Jane Simmonds

Aims

1. To review the role of exercise, rehabilitation and fitness conditioning programmes in the management of JHS and hypermobility
2. To review the tissue changes associated with immobilization, remobilization and reconditioning with reference to hypermobility and JHS
3. To provide the reader with an understanding of the fundamental principles of exercise physiology and training and their applications in devising integrated rehabilitation and fitness programmes for JHS and the hypermobile individual
4. To review the role of hydrotherapy and deep water running in the rehabilitation of JHS
5. To raise and discuss the issues related to injury risk, screening and management strategies pertaining to sport and performance participation of the hypermobile individual

---

INTRODUCTION

Exercise, manual therapy, electrotherapy and education form the basis of the physiotherapy management of neuromusculoskeletal injuries and disorders. Well designed and monitored exercise programmes and participation in appropriate physical activity have been shown repeatedly to be an effective modality for promoting and maintaining long-term physical fitness and health (Bird et al. 1998, Egger et al. 1998).

Few studies have investigated the effectiveness of exercise in individuals with generalized joint laxity and JHS. However, in a study of children diagnosed with JHS, Kerr et al. (2000) report a good response to a daily monitored and modified exercise programme. Likewise, Shoen et al. (1982) report a good response to a generalized progressive exercise programme in adults with JHS. Furthermore, Hinton (1986), in a case study of rehabilitation of multiple joint instability associated with Ehlers–Danlos syndrome, also reports favourable outcomes with exercise. The author's clinical experience indicates that carefully designed and monitored exercise and fitness programmes, in association with lifestyle modification, are effective in the management of patients with this condition. However, exercise should be prescribed with prudence and patience, as the symptoms of JHS can easily be exacerbated.

The physiotherapy management of JHS is complex. Not only is there the challenge of improving static and dynamic joint stability and exercise tolerance, but there may also be the associated problems of chronic pain and fatigue. Hypermobility has been found to be associated with fibromyalgia (FM) (Goldman 1991, Acasuso-Diaz and Collantes-Estevez 1998).

Fibromyalgia is a contentious subject, being described in the literature as a chronic pain condition with unknown aetiology (Wolfe et al. 1990). The symptoms of FM include widespread pain, localized tenderness over specific sites, fatigue, sleep disturbance and morning stiffness. Irritable bowel syndrome and anxiety are also commonly seen (Wolfe et al. 1990). It is diagnosed using the American College of Rheumatology (ACR) diagnostic criteria, which include widespread pain and tenderness on palpation of at least 11 of 18 specified points on the body (Wolfe et al. 1990, Ali 2001a).

In the study by Goldman (1991) of 91 hypermobile patients diagnosed with fibromyalgia, between 79% and 85% displayed significant symptomatic improvements after performing a regular exercise programme. Although Cherpel and Marks (2000) cite criticisms of the study design they comment that it is one of the few investigations into the effects of exercise on individuals with hypermobility and fibromyalgia and its potential for modifying the course of the syndrome.

The subject of chronic pain management is dealt with in detail in Chapter 10. However, it is important to be aware of the association between hypermobility and chronic pain, so as to prevent the deterioration of symptoms to this level of disability and to be able to identify those individuals who would best benefit from a specific pain management programme.

THE PRINCIPLES OF REHABILITATION, HEALTH AND FITNESS

Rehabilitation and fitness reconditioning programmes may be described as dynamic systems of prescribed exercise and activities aimed at reversing and preventing the effects of injury, disease and inactivity. They aim to restore the individual to his or her full health and physical fitness potential.

Health has been redefined as not just a disease-free state, but includes the physical, mental, social, emotional and spiritual state of the individual on a continuum from near death to optimal functioning (Bird et al. 1998). Physical fitness has been described by Lamb (1984) as 'the capacity of the individual to successfully meet the present and potential physical challenges of life and comprises of elements such as flexibility, strength, anaerobic power, speed and aerobic endurance'. The other physical parameters of balance, coordination, speed and muscular endurance may also be added to this definition.

Research has repeatedly demonstrated that regular participation in physical activity benefits all members of the population, regardless of age, gender, or whether they suffer from recognized medical conditions or not (Bird et al. 1998). A summary of these benefits includes:

- Improved quality of life;
- Reduced risk of cardiovascular disease;

- Improved emotional and mental health;
- Improved ability to cope with the demands of life;
- Reduced severity of particular diseases and disorders;
- Minimized effects of ageing;
- Improved physical capacity;
- Assists the socialization process;
- Assists the growth and development of children and adolescents.

Exercise prescription

When designing exercise programmes for rehabilitation purposes the term exercise prescription is commonly used. This implies making an assessment, planning and advocating exercises tailored to meet an individual's needs. It involves understanding the adaptive changes of soft tissue and bone in deconditioned states and during the deconditioning process. In addition, it demands of the physiotherapist an understanding of the laws and principles of exercise physiology and training. In the author's clinical experience, individuals with JHS often present for physiotherapy with multiple joint instabilities and in a deconditioned state. This is usually as a result of recurrent injury, pain and long-term postural misuse.

Joint instability has been suggested to be the underlying cause of microtrauma and subsequent joint and muscle pain in children with JHS (Gedalia and Brewer 1993). It may be further postulated that at least some of the pain experienced in adults with JHS also results from this. Joint stability is determined by the efficient functioning of the neuromusculoskeletal system. Deficiency in any of these systems resulting from inflammatory disease, trauma or neural impairment compromises stability (Kerr et al. 2000). Understanding the neuromusculoskeletal adaptive changes to immobilization and inactivity in relationship to joint stability is then of particular clinical significance to the management of hypermobility and JHS.

Panjabi's (1992) theories provide us with a good model for understanding spinal instability.

This theory stimulates thought into the relationship between hypermobility and instability of the spine and other joints.

TISSUE RESPONSE TO IMMOBILIZATION AND INACTIVITY

Bone

The equilibrium of bone absorption and accretion is maintained by weight-bearing and muscular contraction. The rate of bone cell turnover decreases after 10–15 days of immobilization. Loss of bone density is evidenced by a loss of the normal trabecular pattern. The mechanical properties of bone, including elastic resistance and hardness, steadily decline with increased duration of immobilization (Burdeaux and Hutchinson 1953, Hardt 1972, Landry and Fleisch 1964). After 12 weeks of immobilization bone hardness is reduced by 55–60% of normal. Most of these losses are recoverable by muscle contraction and weight-bearing in a comparable period of time (Steinberg 1980).

Muscle

The effects of immobilization and inactivity on muscle have been thoroughly investigated and include a decrease in fibre size, changes in sarcomere alignment and configuration and reduced muscle mass (Booth 1987, Harrelson 1998, MacDougall et al. 1977).

Mitochondria are also reduced in number, size and function and, together with the histochemical changes that occur with immobilization, result in a reduction in the oxidative capacity of muscle (Booth 1987, Booth and Kelso 1973, MacDougall et al. 1977). This increases the fatiguability of muscles. Reduction in muscle endurance has been shown to occur as early as 7 days post immobilization (Rifenberick and Max 1974). Atrophy occurs in both fast twitch (type I) and slow twitch (type II) muscle fibres; however, it is generally accepted that there is greater degeneration in slow twitch fibres (Harrelson 1998). The rate of muscle atrophy is greatest in the first 5–7 days of the immobilization period, after which the rate of loss slows down significantly (Booth 1987).

Muscle atrophy resulting from immobilization appears to be selective. Muscles also atrophy as a result of reflex inhibition due to pain, fear of pain, injury and inflammation (Harrelson 1998).

Nerve

Few changes in neural structures have been identified as being due to immobilization. The neurodynamic function of muscle spindles, articular mechanoreceptors, motor efferents and sensory afferents are difficult to assess experimentally. Empirical data, however, suggest that there is a neural reflex causing muscle atrophy that results from joint damage and immobilization (Engles 1994, Harrelson 1998).

Connective tissue

The effects of immobilization on connective tissue have also been studied extensively. Studies on rabbit knees by Akeson et al. (1980) showed changes in collagen, glycosaminoglycans (GAG) and water content. It was also observed that the connective tissue, when immobilized, appeared 'woody' rather than glistening, and this they believed was due to water loss. Theories regarding the pathomechanics of joint contracture suggested that the loss of water and GAG increased the space between the collagen fibres, altering the amount of free movement between fibres. This lack of movement made the tissue less elastic, less plastic and more brittle, the implication being that capsular structures, including ligaments, would fail at lower loads after periods of immobilization.

Ligament

In addition to the connective tissue changes mentioned above, specific changes in ligaments

as a result of immobilization have been documented. Ligaments remodel as a response to mechanical stress, becoming stronger and stiffer when subject to loading. A study on the anterior cruciate ligaments of rats revealed that inactivity and rest resulted in weaker, more compliant tissue (Cabaud et al. 1980). Studies performed on dogs and primates suggest that the alterations in the mechanical properties of ligaments are a result of increased osteoclastic activity at the bone–ligament junction, rather than actual ligament atrophy (Laros 1971, Noyes et al. 1974). These alterations lead to a decrease in tensile strength and reduce the ability of ligaments to provide joint stability.

CLINICAL IMPLICATIONS OF IMMOBILIZATION

Bone that has undergone local osteoporosis after fracture or immobilization is less able to bear weight or withstand the normal forces of compression, tension and shear. Due care must be taken when using manual techniques and exercise to joints and limbs that have undergone immobilization. It may be postulated that in the case of JHS, inactivity due to pain may increase the risk of osteoporosis, particularly in postmenopausal women. This is another area requiring further research.

Immobilization and inactivity of muscles result in weakness owing to loss of muscle mass. In addition, muscle stiffness occurs with the laying down of irregular cross-linked connective tissue. Postural slow twitch muscles fibres crossing one joint tend to atrophy the fastest (Engles 1994). This will be evidenced in activities requiring sustained or repeated muscle contraction, i.e. standing, sitting and walking. Such changes also contribute to joint instability which, as mentioned earlier, is a common feature in JHS. Rehabilitation initially should focus on developing the endurance and strength of the local postural antigravity muscles.

It has been suggested that abnormality of collagen synthesis is the pathogenic root of JHS (Child 1986). If this already fragile connective tissue is further compromised in terms of strength and stiffness as a result of immobilization, inactivity and deconditioning, it could have a major impact on joint stability for individuals with hypermobility.

Changes in the muscle and connective tissues, in addition to alterations of neurodynamic function that occur as a result of deconditioning and immobilization, may provide some explanation of why, in clinical practice, we observe individuals with JHS who have become inactive because of pain or injury often displaying considerable joint instability, reduced muscle strength, endurance, poor proprioception and vulnerability to injury.

TISSUE RESPONSE TO REMOBILIZATION AND REACTIVATION

Most studies investigating the response of bone and soft tissue to mobilization have looked primarily at normal subjects. Muscles begin to regenerate within 3–5 days of the start of a reconditioning programme (Cooper 1972, Zarins 1982). Within the first week, muscle weight increases. Witzmann et al. (1982) report that muscle strength can be regained by 6 weeks of exercise; however, normal muscle weight may not be fully achieved until 3 months.

Recovery of bone, nerve and connective tissue occurs at a much slower rate than that of muscle, largely because of the extensive vascular supply of muscle tissue. Connective tissue is the slowest to return to normal after injury. Ligaments begin to regain tensile strength by the fifth week of reconditioning after injury. A healing ligament may take between 6 months and 3 years to recover fully, depending on the severity of the injury (Tipton et al. 1970). Thus, although stressing connective tissues in the recovery phase is necessary, it needs to be done with great caution. Moderate-frequency low-intensity endurance exercises have been shown to have a beneficial effect on the mechanical properties of ligaments. It has been suggested that such exercises may result in increased collagen production and hypertrophy of fibre bundles. This claim is supported by the work of Cabaud et al. (1980) and Williams et al. (1988). Non-weight bearing isometric exercises, although helpful, are no substitute for the stimulation of weight-bearing and loading (Harrelson 1998).

It is of particular interest that in many studies the effect of regular exercise and mechanical stress had the beneficial effect of increasing the mass of ligaments and tendons, rendering them stiffer and able to tolerate heavier loads at failure. Microscopic examination showed, among other changes, an increase in the size of collagen fibrils (Woo et al. 1982). Future research investigating the tissue response of collagen-defective tissue to exercise will be important in understanding and prescribing exercises for individuals with connective tissue disorders.

APPLIED PRINCIPLES OF REHABILITATION AND TRAINING

In order to design truly holistic and integrated rehabilitation and fitness programmes for hypermobile individuals, both the physical and psychological aspects need to be considered and addressed. The physical components of a programme include paced and monitored training to improve:

- Proprioception, coordination and kinaesthesia;
- Core stability endurance and strength;
- Global muscle strength and endurance;
- Controlled flexibility;
- Cardiovascular fitness;
- Relaxation and breathing.

In addition to the above, visualization techniques may be taught to help reduce pain and promote healing. Advice on diet, adequate rest and pacing is also important. The importance of rest should not be underestimated, as it is only during deep sleep that the muscles fully relax. When sleep is disturbed muscles fatigue (Ali 2001b). Exercise classes and the use of music may also assist motivation and compliance.

Principles of exercise physiology and training

Knowledge and application of the principles of exercise physiology and training are essential for the physiotherapist in designing effective programmes. These principles were originally developed by exercise physiologists to provide effective guidelines for athletic and sports training. They have been adapted and used by those involved with rehabilitation to optimize recovery after injury, disease and immobilization. The classic text by Rasche and Burke (1977) discusses the principles in detail. Harrelson and Leaver-Dunn (1998) include an excellent section on the principles of training in relation to sports rehabilitation. There follows a summary and discussion of the main principles and how they may be applied to the rehabilitation in JHS and hypermobility.

Readiness principle

This can be understood to be the preparedness of an individual to undertake an exercise programme. This principle originally applied to athletes recommencing fitness training after acute injury or lay-off, and may also be applied to the rehabilitation situation. For example, in clinical practice it is often necessary for a patient with JHS to have their pain moderated first by medication and/or other therapeutic means before they are able to undertake a programme of exercise. It is equally important that the patient feels psychologically prepared and committed before commencing the programme.

Overload and progression principles

Beneficial human performance adaptations occur as a response to stress applied at levels beyond a certain threshold, but within certain limits of tolerance and safety. Low levels of stress to which the body has already adapted are not sufficient to induce a further training response. In the **useful** range – i.e. where the stress is above the threshold – an adequate training response may cause some disruption of tissue and change in biomechanical balance. During the period between bouts of exercise, repair and restoration occur, after which an adaptation takes place in the tissue, raising the individual's stress threshold to a higher level. Because of the underlying defective collagen in the connective tissue of the hypermobile individual, it is important to be prudent when prescribing exercise, particularly with reference to increasing the number of repetitions and resistance. Stress is required to achieve strength or endurance gains; however, if the threshold of a hypermobile individual is stressed too much and too early, beyond a certain limit, there may be danger of symptom exacerbation and injury.

Specificity

Exercise, whether aimed at improving cardiovascular function, proprioception or strength, needs to be targeted at specific systems and activities. For example, if one of the aims of a programme is to improve cardiovascular endurance, then the prescribed exercise needs to involve the large muscle groups and be performed for a minimum of 2–3 minutes in order to stimulate cardiac function and the aerobic energy system. Furthermore, if long-distance rowing is an objective, then training the endurance capacity and functional actions of the muscle groups involved in rowing is also necessary.

Strength development in particular is known to be highly specific (Rasche and Burke 1977). Strength can be divided into three discrete groups: dynamic strength, which is the ability to move or support the weight of the body repeatedly over a given period; static strength, which is the ability to exert a maximum force continuously for a brief period; and explosive strength, which is the ability to exert maximum energy in one short burst (Rasche and Burke 1977). In the case of hypermobility the development of both dynamic and static strength is important for the development of joint stability. Therefore, when planning a programme of exercises specific types of strength training need to be considered.

Explosive strength applies particularly to sporting situations and should be specifically trained for should it be required, such as in performing leaps in ballet, or kicking in football.

Intensity and frequency

Training needs to be sufficiently spaced to allow tissue growth, nutritional replenishment and biochemical resynthesis to take place. However, it needs to be frequent enough to provide for neurophysiological change (Rasche and Burke 1977). There are implications here for the JHS patient, as clinically the author has found that recovery time after exercise is slow and the training response reduced. This may be due to lactic acid build-up and reduced oxidative functioning of the muscles. Therefore, spacing exercises throughout the day and adequate rest is important. Further investigation into this area is clearly required.

ASSESSING AND DESIGNING EXERCISE PROGRAMMES FOR JHS

The problem-solving approach is the logical way to tackle the challenge of designing rehabilitation programmes. The assessment is crucial for identifying and prioritizing the problems to be addressed. A word of caution is necessary. When assessing patients with JHS, symptom irritability is frequently high and often leads to an exacerbation of pain later. Questioning with regard to this is important, and the objective assessment may need to be performed over several days.

Subjective assessment

The subjective examination includes collecting information regarding age, race, gender, working status, stress levels, and a current and past medical and family history. It also includes questions relating to current and past physical activity tolerance and preferred modes of exercise. It is important to ask detailed questions relating to functional ability on good and bad days. This is helpful in determining the baseline functional level for the programme. An evaluation of current pain levels using a simple visual analogue scale (0–10) can be used. Alternatively, the short McGill Pain Questionnaire can be helpful (Melzack 1987). Questions relating to general health, diet, medication, ergonomics at work and in the home should be included, along with 24-hour pain behaviour and aggravating factors. Enquiring about support from family and work colleagues should also be included in the assessment.

Objective assessment

The objective assessment consists of documentable physical findings that the physiotherapist discovers through observation, inspection, palpation, muscle, joint, cardiovascular and neurophysiological testing.

Observation

Observation of gait and general physical attitude are made at the initial meeting with the patient and during the subjective evaluation. The evaluation of posture, both dynamic and static, is of particular importance, as the impact of several hypermobile joints on the kinetic chain is substantial. Posture and gait analysis may be examined by direct observation or by photographic and video documentation. These types of visual feedback system are excellent for patient education and monitoring progress.

When assessing posture and gait, it can also be helpful to request the patient to report areas of muscle tension, pain and stiffness. In addition, information about proprioceptive and kinaesthetic sensations, such as asymmetries between sides, variations in sensations of heaviness and lightness in the limbs during standing, walking and sitting to standing, is useful. This is particularly important when assessing hypermobile individuals, as proprioception has been found to be altered (Hall et al. 1995, Mallik 1994).

Functional active range of motion and muscle testing

The quality and range of movement should be assessed, observing both the recruitment and the timing of muscle contractions. These elements affect static and dynamic joint stability, both of which in the author's clinical experience are frequently impaired when individuals are requested to perform activities without locking their joints and 'hanging on their ligaments'.

The assessment of the individual's ability to sustain static joint position and postures is also crucial. This ability is largely determined by the degree of ligament laxity, muscle tone, static strength, proprioceptive ability and endurance capability of the muscles (Harrelson 1998). Specific static and dynamic muscle testing of core trunk muscles, in particular transversus abdominis, multifidus and the deep neck flexors, can be evaluated and trained using pressure biofeedback, palpation and muscle re-education techniques. Readers are referred to the work of Hodges and Richardson (1996), Hides et al. (1994), Jull (2001) and O'Sullivan et al. (1997).

Manual muscle testing as recommended by Kendall et al. (1983) may also be used. Other global and peripheral muscle groups should also be assessed in functional positions, i.e. testing the ability to sustain a neutral joint position in weight bearing (e.g. the knee or lumbar spine on standing) can also be useful in gauging functional isometric strength and endurance, particularly in a hypermobile individual who may have adopted the habit of 'hanging on their ligaments'.

Proprioception and kinaesthesia

The subject of proprioception deserves special attention when discussing the rehabilitation of hypermobile individuals. The component of neuromuscular control necessary for joint stability is very important in a rehabilitation programme (Harrelson and Leaver-Dunn 1998), and even more in the case of the JHS population, where there are known deficits.

'Proprioception is considered a specialized variation of the sensory modality of touch and encompasses the sensations of joint movement (kinaesthesia) and joint position (joint position sense)' (Lephart 1992). Both conscious and unconscious proprioception are considered to be important for efficient and safe joint movement and stability (Lephart et al. 1994).

The ligaments play a very important role in joint proprioception. This has been documented by many authors, including Kennedy et al. (1982) and Schultz et al. (1984). Reflex muscular contractions occur when the Golgi receptors, located in the ligaments, are stimulated by abnormal stress. In addition to the contribution of the joint capsule receptors, Harrelson and Leaver-Dunn (1998) cite the important discovery by Skinner et al. (1986), who investigated patients who had undergone knee arthroplasty. They observed that the deep receptors in the muscle spindle, Golgi tendon organs and pain and pressure receptors make a significant contribution to joint stabilization. Finally, it has been suggested that the mechanoreceptors (Ruffini, Meissner's and Pacinian corpuscles), thermoreceptors and nociceptors found in the skin also play a significant role in proprioception (Table 8.1) (Willis and Grossman 1981). This may be an interesting finding in relation to JHS, as hyperextensibility of skin may eventually be found to play a role in altered proprioception and kinaesthetic sense.

Assessment of proprioception, kinaesthesia and coordination

Subjective and objective evaluations of proprioception, kinaesthesia and coordination can be assessed using a battery of tests. Objective laboratory testing is available for some measurements; however, clinical proprioceptive and kinaesthetic testing validation is still in its infancy. Balance exercises are the most commonly used as subjective testing procedures for the lower limb and

Table 8.1   Summary of the location and function of the mechanoreceptors

Location	Receptor	Function
Joint capsule	Ruffini's corpuscle	Sensitive to articular pressure changes Monitors amplitude and velocity of joint position change Monitors the speed and direction of capsular stretch
Joint capsule	Pacinian corpuscle	Activated by the onset and cessation of joint movement Monitors changes in joint acceleration and deceleration
Joint capsule	Golgi–Mazzoni corpuscle	Monitors compression of the joint capsule
Joint capsule	Golgi–ligament ending	Sensitive to tension and stretch of ligaments
Joint capsule	Free nerve endings	Slowly adapting pain receptor
Musculotendinous junction	Golgi–tendon organ	Monitors the stretch and contraction of the musculotendinous junction
Muscle belly	Muscle spindle	Monitors muscle length and rate of change of muscle length
Skin	Free nerve endings	Monitors temperature and pain
Skin	Meissner's corpuscles Pacinian corpuscles Ruffini's corpuscles	Mechanoreceptors

(Modified from Harrelson and Leaver-Dunn 1998, Willis and Grossman 1981, Kennedy et al. 1982, Schultz et al. 1984, Skinner et al. 1986).

trunk proprioception. Guiskiewicz and Perrin (1996) have described a number of these, including the following subjective observations of postural sway (Rhomberg's test), one-legged standing (stork test) and tandem Rhomberg's test, which requires the placement of one foot in front of the other, heel to toe. In the case of the hypermobile individual it is important that joint position is noted, as these individuals will commonly lock their joints for stability. The author has found subjective observations of dynamic balance on rocker boards, half rolls and line walking useful in highlighting balance and coordination problems. In addition to these tests other subjective observations of the patient's ability to reposition a joint or body part can give the physiotherapist useful feedback regarding their body awareness and kinaesthetic sense. Frequently the hypermobile individual is observed to overshoot when tested. These tests, performed in supine, sitting, standing and functional positions, require validation.

Neurological evaluation

Evaluation of the neural system structures may be necessary, and includes testing the mobility of the nervous system (Butler 1991) dermatome sensation, deep tendon reflexes and motor function.

Functional capacity, cardiovascular and morphological measures

An assessment would not be complete without an evaluation of cardiovascular function, or at least functional capacity. As discussed earlier, a comprehensive rehabilitation plan should include global aerobic fitness measures. Baseline measures of blood pressure and resting heart rate need to be taken routinely. The author has found low blood pressure to be a frequent clinical finding in JHS. This has been confirmed to be due to autonomic dysfunction (Gazit et al. 2003). Low blood pressure resulting in dizziness should be investigated and monitored before any strenuous exercise is advocated. Any suggestion of cardiac or respiratory problems from the medical history should be thoroughly explored, as mitral valve pathologies may occasionally be associated with vascular-type Ehlers–Danlos (EDS IV) and Marfan syndromes (Grahame 2000a). Asthma and wheezing have also been found to be associated with JHS (Morgan et al. 1996).

Cardiovascular function, functional capacity and walking ability can be assessed using a number of tests. The choice will depend on age, current disability and health. For older, less able individuals the 3-minute walk test as described by Worsford and Simpson (2001) may be used.

The 10-metre increment shuttle walk test as described by MacSween et al. (2001) is a useful baseline indicator of aerobic capacity.

For the fitter individual, the 3- or 5-minute step test, the 6–12-minute walk test, the physical work capacity (PWC) 170 bike test and treadmill gas exchange tests can be utilized. The American College of Sports Medicine 1980 and 1988 has produced two very good resources for exercise testing guidelines.

Body weight, girth measurements, height and percentage body fat may also be measured and documented to complete the morphological clinical picture.

ANALYSIS AND DEVELOPMENT OF THE REHABILITATION PROGRAMME

Following the examination and identification of a specific problems list, the rehabilitation programme can be designed. At this point it is a good idea for physiotherapist and patient to develop realistic short-, medium- and long-term goals. These may include strength and endurance gains, personal independence, weight loss, a return to sport and a return to work. It is also important at this point to spend time educating the patient about the nature of the condition, the rationale behind the approach to rehabilitation and the need for compliance with exercise, pacing of activities, lifestyle modification, responsibility and joint care.

The rehabilitation programme aims should be directed towards modulating the pain, improving proprioception and kinaesthetic sense, achieving and maintaining static and dynamic neuromuscular joint stability, balance and control. It should also aim to improve general muscular endurance, cardiovascular function, general health and wellbeing. Box 8.1 provides a summary of these stages.

Rehabilitation

In the very early stages of rehabilitation emphasis should be placed on improving body awareness,

---

Box 8.1 Summary of rehabilitation stages

Early stage
Education regarding nature of the condition
Pain management and discussion of management plan
Joint position and kinaesthetic awareness, local spinal and proximal joint-stabilizing exercises
Breathing and relaxation exercises
Commence gait and posture awareness exercises
Introduce gentle PNF rhythmic stabilizations, Swiss ball exercises for proprioception, dynamic balance, coordination and strength development
Hydrotherapy

Middle stage
Introduce global and peripheral joint muscle strength, endurance and controlled relative flexibility training
Introduce relative flexibility exercises
Hydrotherapy
Focus on dynamic balance and coordination exercises using Swiss ball, hydrotherapy, proprioception boards and roll boards and rolls
Commence low-level cardiovascular training; walking, water walking

Late stage
Increase functional cardiovascular exercise training, deep-water running, walking and Nordic track
Continue and progress relative flexibility exercises
Progress static and dynamic muscle and endurance strength training using theraband, pulley, hand weights, body weight and gym equipment

Final stage
Rehabilitation focuses on functional rehabilitation specific to set outcome goals and development of long-term fitness maintenance programmes. Pilates, yoga, Tai chi, Qi Gong and Feldenkrais are good examples of exercise programmes that may be useful for maintaining condition

---

proprioceptive and proximal joint stability. Muscle strengthening and endurance exercises may include isometric and joint proprioception exercises in pain-free positions, and gradually progressing to functional positions (Fig. 8.1).

Proprioceptive neuromuscular facilitation (PNF) techniques may also be used to facilitate muscle co-contraction and neuromuscular recruitment. Rhythmic stabilizations and joint approximation techniques around the pelvis, scapular area and neck can be used in sitting, four-point kneeling, standing, and in combination with the Swiss ball (Fig. 8.2).

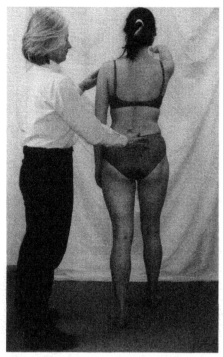

Figure 8.1   Activation of the multifidus muscle in stride standing

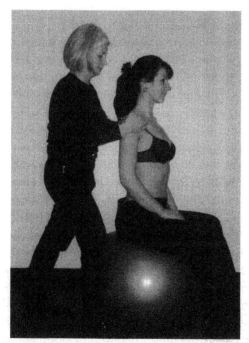

Figure 8.2   Rhythmic stabilization around the shoulder girdle. This can be performed on a Swiss ball to increase trunk stability

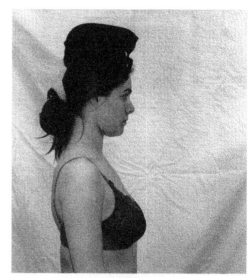

Figure 8.3   Functional stability and strength exercise for neck

A functional exercise that has also been found to be beneficial for cervical spine stabilization and training the neck muscles in JHS is to have the individual sit with a weighted rice bag on the head, gradually increasing the length of sitting time and the weight of the bag (Taylor, S. 2001, personal communication) (Fig. 8.3).

Later in the programme balance and rocker boards, half rolls and sit-fit cushions can be utilized in functional positions of standing, sitting and kneeling so as to make training as specific to function as possible.

The Swiss ball is very popular as an exercise tool. Patients with JHS find it comfortable, challenging and therapeutic. Swiss ball techniques as described by Carrière (1998) can be used creatively to improve kinaesthetic and proprioceptive sense and muscle strength, to reduce spasm and to control movement by activating the reticular formation and the reticulospinal pathways. Exercises may start with postural work in sitting, gently bouncing on the ball to stimulate the vestibular system. More advanced exercises to help pelvic control and core stability can be prescribed as progressions (Fig. 8.4).

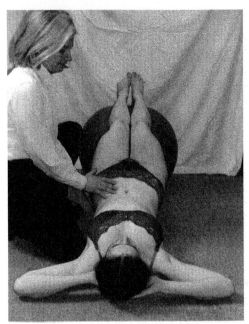

Figure 8.4 Bridging on the Swiss ball can help improve trunk stability

Once a degree of trunk and local joint stability has been achieved, individuals should be encouraged to perform exercises in more dynamic activities. In the author's opinion walking should be particularly encouraged, as it is a highly functional integrated exercise that promotes proprioception, co-contraction and reflex postural stability through the joint approximation of weight-bearing. Individuals can be instructed to focus on recruiting the transversus abdominis, multifidus and lower and middle fibres of trapezius, to reinforce their other specific stabilizing exercises.

As the rehabilitation programme progresses, exercises can be made more challenging and dynamic using resistive exercise tubing and light weights. The number of repetitions and exercises performed should be based on assessment of fatigue and the ability to maintain the correct **form** of the activity. The principles of training should be applied to the exercise prescription, i.e. when aiming to improve muscular endurance and activate slow twitch fibres, the number of repetitions and length of contraction should be high, while the resistance remains relatively low.

Flexibility

Controlled, supported stretching may be prescribed for tight tissues. Clinically, the author has found that individuals with JHS frequently find stretching relieves the sensations of stiffness and discomfort. Short stiff muscles which result from malalignments and altered recruitment patterns may be addressed using PNF exercises and the relative flexibility approach described and demonstrated by Sahrmann (2002). The author cautions once again that stretching should be very carefully controlled, as the hypermobile joints and more pliable muscles tend to move and possibly overstretch before the tighter tissues, and may sometimes aggravate symptoms.

Cardiovascular exercise

Cardiovascular exercise can be instituted once proximal stability has been addressed. Walking, cycling, Nordic track, swimming and deep-water running are all useful. Finding the aerobic exercise that an individual enjoys is very important as this will aid compliance.

A direct linear relationship between heart rate and oxygen consumption occurs when exercising at between 40% and 90% of maximum heart rate. Cardiovascular training is believed to be optimal at somewhere between 60% and 90% of an individual's maximum heart rate. Lower level aerobic activity – around 50% – is usually prescribed when weight loss is required. Karvonen's Law (Egger et al. 1998) is frequently used to calculate a training heart rate. This formula uses the individual's resting heart rate, training percentage and maximum heart rate (220 – age) to obtain a training target heart rate. For example, a 40-year-old wishing to train at 70% of maximum heart rate with a resting heart rate of 72 would need to achieve a target heart rate of 147.6 beats per minute [(180 – 72)(70 + 72)]. This formula, and others like it, has been developed and used for normal healthy populations by exercise physiologists and sports scientists for several decades. However, prescriptions for exercise for other members of society need to be carefully designed and made specific to the individual, taking into consideration each person's current state of fitness, the presence of disease, age, sex, altitude, temperature, medication and motivation.

In the clinical situation it may be useful to calculate maximum heart rate and target heart rates in the very late stages of rehabilitation of a person hoping to return to sport. However, in the earlier phases of reconditioning programmes these formulae are not always applicable. For example, in the case of JHS more intense levels of exercise may lead to fatigue and result in poor dynamic neuromuscular control, further muscle imbalance, and possibly injury and pain.

Probably the safest and best method of prescribing cardiovascular exercise is by evaluating the individual's response to an exercise programme and asking for verbal feedback on perceived levels of exhaustion. This can be done by having the individual exercise performed with the therapist monitoring the response. For example, the exercise prescribed may be slow walking for 10–15 minutes. This distance can be gradually increased as the individual is able; likewise the speed can be increased. The minimum frequency of aerobic training needs to be three to four times per week. Clinically, in the case of JHS sufferers the author has found that daily, or almost daily, low-intensity exercise is the most beneficial.

Varying the mode of exercise between walking, stationary cycling, swimming and deep-water walking or running is helpful for both motivation and reducing the strain on various joints and tissues.

The cardiovascular effects of exercise conditioning have been well documented. In untrained deconditioned individuals oxygen consumption levels can be expected to improve by between 10% and 30% over a 3–6-month period (Irwin 1994). The amount of improvement depends on many variables, including the state of fitness before exercise, the intensity and duration of training, age, and the presence of systemic pathology (Irwin 1994). The best results are achieved

when the training heart rate exceeds 60% of maximal heart rate. It should also be noted here that low-level aerobic exercise is also helpful for weight loss.

Training diaries can be useful for aiding exercise compliance, recording improvements, and for noting exercises or activities that either relieve or aggravate pain.

Final stages of rehabilitation and preventative fitness programmes

Towards the latter stages of rehabilitation, cardiovascular exercise can be increased by up to between 60% and 80% of maximum heart rate. Attention to dynamic posture should continue to be emphasized. Light weights, exercise bands and gym equipment can be used to improve strength and endurance. Climbing, an activity which requires the use of both the upper and lower limb stabilizers, has been found anecdotally to be helpful in improving dynamic core stability and integrated coordination. Vleeming's sling theory may support this suggestion (Vleeming et al. 1995). Further investigation is clearly required to validate the use of such activities.

For individuals wishing to return to active sport, specific functional rehabilitation is crucial. Many individuals with generalized joint hypermobility find yoga, swimming, Pilates, Feldenkrais, Tai Chi and Qi Gong helpful in maintaining general health and dynamic strength and controlled flexibility.

The time frame for rehabilitation of individuals varies according to the severity of the condition, the level of deconditioning and commitment to the programme. Frequently, individuals with JHS need to be supervised and monitored for between 6 months and 2 years.

HYDROTHERAPY

Hydrotherapy is popular with individuals with JHS. The combination of buoyancy, support and warmth makes it a very conducive arena for exercise. As well as being a medium for achieving physical goals, hydrotherapy has added psychological and social benefits (Skinner and Thomson 1993, Petajan et al. 1996). The reduction in sympathetic activity that occurs as a result of buoyancy may alter tone, diminish pain and spasm and achieve relaxation. Sensory stimulus provided by turbulence can increase body awareness (Hurley and Turner 1991, Mano et al. 1985, Fuller 1998). The three-dimensional resistive environment, combined with the viscosity of the water, aids kinaesthetic sense and improves the synchronization of motor unit contractions through the whole range of joint movement (Fuller 1998).

Bad Ragaz techniques, as described by Davis and Harrison (1988), rhythmic stabilizations, isometrics, slow walking and carefully controlled active exercises using open and closed chain movements are particularly helpful for developing core stability in the early and middle stages of rehabilitation. Exercises can be progressed using turbulence, webbed gloves and weights to increase resistance.

Once trunk and proximal stability has been taught, deep-water walking and running with the aid of a buoyancy vest can be used to improve coordination and cardiovascular fitness. This form of aerobic exercise training is particularly popular with JHS sufferers as they are often able to exercise for longer without exacerbating their symptoms (Fig. 8.5). Water immersion has the added advantage of improving the circulation of blood to working muscles, which enhances oxygen supply and aids the removal of carbon dioxide and lactic acid (Fuller 1998). It is also a potent diuretic, natriuretic and kaluretic, which may explain some of the perceived benefits (Grahame et al. 1978).

Deep-water running should **not** be undertaken in overheated hydrotherapy pools because of the risk of hyperthermia, and may be commenced with as little as 5 minutes. Speed and distance can then be gradually increased as tolerated, applying the principles used for cardiovascular training.

HYPERMOBILITY, SPORT AND PERFORMANCE

Flexibility is an important physical fitness parameter in sport and in the performing arts. The combination of flexibility, neuromuscular control, dynamic coordination and rhythm is essential for most sporting and athletic performances. In particular, gymnastics, ballet and dance, circus performance and diving require a high degree of flexibility. Grahame and Jenkins (1972) suggest that hypermobility may be viewed as an asset in ballet.

It has been suggested that individuals with hypermobile joints incur a wide variety of traumatic and overuse lesions, internal joint derangements, such as dislocations and subluxations, and recurrent joint effusions, arthralgia, or myalgias which lead them to seek medical attention (Cherpel and Marks 1999). Tarsal and carpal tunnel syndromes, reflex sympathetic dystrophy and sciatica may also be associated with the condition, (Grahame 1971, Beighton et al. 1989, Francis et al. 1987, Grahame et al. 1981). Keller et al. (1987) have contentiously stated that 'there is no evidence to suggest that physiological laxity is associated with any increase in injury rate'.

There is mixed opinion as to whether individuals with widespread hypermobility should be advised against competitive and elite participation

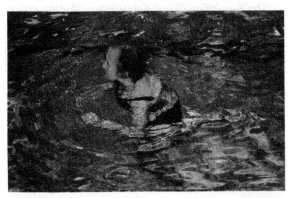

Figure 8.5 Deep-water running

in sport because of the risk of injury and the long-term joint damage. Klemp and Learmouth (1984) found that hypermobile dancers sustained more injuries than the controls. Kirby et al. (1981) found that gymnasts who had a greater toe-touching ability also experienced low back discomfort. A number of studies (Ekstrand and Gillquist 1983, Nicholas 1970) have documented that footballers who have specific ligamentous instability have a higher risk of injury. A study of secondary-school athletes did not find any relationship between ligament laxity and injury rates (Grana and Moretz 1985). This finding was supported by Decoster et al. (1979) in a study of lacrosse players. Steiner (1987) concluded that inherited knee joint hypermobility played little role in the causes of most knee injuries, with the exception of patellar dislocation. One of the most significant findings was made by Lysens et al. (1989), who discovered that ligament laxity in combination with muscle tightness and lower limb malalignment was a significant risk factor in overuse sports injuries.

Vincenzo (1995) has contentiously suggested that **instability** rather than hypermobility is the risk factor that pertains to sport. The author challenges this notion on the basis of mounting evidence that hypermobility predisposes to instability, particularly in sports where repetitive, high-load, explosive ballistic unilateral actions

are involved, such as in tennis, golf, baseball pitching and kicking. It would seem prudent for hypermobile individuals to avoid contact sports. Future epidemiological research will provide clarity in this area.

Individuals with marked joint laxity, Ehlers–Danlos and Marfan syndromes should be screened for cardiorespiratory abnormality before undertaking strenuous physical activity. Hypermobility may also incur other risks related to tissue fragility (Grahame 2000a, b). Easy bruising, poor wound healing and hernias are common clinical findings, and sports physiotherapists and trainers need to be aware of these clinical implications with regard to treatment following sprains, strains and contusions. Advice regarding correctly fitting footwear may be given, and orthotics may be used to correct pes planus and lower limb alignment.

Pre-season screening for hypermobility and joint instability is advisable for children, adolescents and adults participating in competitive sport and performance activities. The presence of generalized joint hypermobility, instability, muscle imbalance, malalignment, the age and gender of the individual, skill level, personality type and the demands of the sport or performance should all be considered when determining an individual's suitability.

Case study

A 35-year-old woman diagnosed with JHS was referred initially to physiotherapy for assessment and management. The areas of pain included constant bilateral, lateral and posterior hip pain, worse on the left, intermittent bilateral knee pain, and left-sided cervicothoracic pain referring into the left upper arm and anterior pectoral region.

Following manual therapy, postural and initial core stability training, she was referred for functional rehabilitation and fitness training.

Medical history revealed that she had performed gymnastics and contortionist tricks in her youth. She scored 5/9 on the Beighton scale, and outside the scale her shoulders, cervical spine, proximal and distal interphalangeal joints were considered hypermobile. She regularly sprained her ankles, and had complained of knee pain since the age of 13. There was also a history of previous back and neck pain and recurrent shoulder capsulitis. She bruised easily,

had poor skin healing and significant fatigue. There was a family history of marfanoid habitus in her brother, both parents and maternal grandfather, although she did not display those features herself. She had anaemia, for which she took iron tablets, and had symptoms of irritable bowel and asthma.

Significant examination findings at the time of referral for rehabilitation

Symptoms had improved with initial physiotherapy of manual therapy and initial core stability exercises. Although her pain could still be severe (8 on a 0–10 scale on bad days), it had become intermittent. She complained of approximately 4 bad days in a fortnight, and this varied between pain in the thoracic, lumbar spine, hips and knees. Spinal pain was provoked by positions sustained for 20 minutes or more, and was worse during periods of increased physical and emotional stress. The knee pain was aggravated by walking, particularly up and down hills. Flare-ups in the neck or hip region were occurring approximately once every month to 6 weeks and could last for a week to 10 days. She complained of generalized weakness on the left side of her body and 'clumsiness'.

She was in full-time employment in a sedentary management position. Office ergonomics were perceived as good, and stress levels were perceived as moderate to high. Her general health had improved over the 5 months that she had been receiving treatment and she was generally less tired. She enjoyed physical activity and was attending a low-level yoga class two to three times per week, which she enjoyed and found relaxing, although it sometimes aggravated her low back symptoms. On a 'good day' she was able to walk 1–2 miles on flat ground without ill effect. She found that hill walking exacerbated her knee pain after a short time. On 'bad days' she found walking difficult.

She complained of some morning stiffness, although this was relieved during the day after gentle activity, but could be made worse with long periods of sustained sitting or excessive activity.

Examination showed that she stood with a posterior pelvic tilt and anteriorly positioned glenohumeral joints, reduced thoracic kyphosis, and slightly hyperextended knees. There was visible bilateral reduction in gluteal tone and bulk. She stood 5' 8" tall and weighed 10 stone. Blood pressure and resting heart rate were within the normal range. The active range of spinal movements was generally good, but cervical side flexion, thoracic rotation, extension and lumbar side flexion showed signs of instability and poor recruitment patterns.

Transversus abdominis and multifidus were weak, but she could isolate and maintain a static contraction. Lower trapezius and both gluteus maximus and medius muscles were also weak, fatigued early, and recruitment and timing were poor (left more than right). The patient could stand on her left leg for 10 seconds with eyes open and for 3–5 seconds with the eyes closed. On the right side the patient was able to stand for 20 seconds with eyes open and for 10 seconds with eyes closed. There was noticeable pelvic instability on this activity.

On joint positioning relocation tests of the pelvis and knees she demonstrated less accuracy on the left, often overshooting joint position and markers. On a mark relocating test, with toe-to-floor markers, the patient was again less accurate, often overshooting with the left foot.

Rehabilitation programme
The agreed short- and long-term aims were:
- To reduce the frequency of flare-ups and pain;
- To improve general health, fitness and functional capacity in order to resume hill walking. Estimated distances of ~4–5 miles;
- To improve muscle balance in order to gain symmetry;

- To improve balance, coordination and kinaesthetic sense in order to reduce 'clumsiness'.

Rehabilitation objectives and plan
To design and develop a daily exercise programme specifically aimed at:
- Improving sitting, standing and dynamic posture;
- Improving dynamic stability and symmetry of the lumbosacral region, neck and shoulder girdle;
- Improving general body awareness and proprioception and kinaesthetic sense of the proximal spine and proximal joints;
- Improving the endurance capacity of local postural and antigravity muscles;
- Increasing the strength of the global trunk and proximal joint muscles;
- Improving cardiovascular endurance and functional capacity.

The rehabilitation programme
The rehabilitation programme consisted of four elements:
- A cardiovascular walking programme that was incorporated into her travel to and from work;
- Graduated Swiss ball proprioceptive and dynamic strengthening exercises in sitting, prone and supine, with legs supported by the ball;
- Dynamic stabilizing and strengthening exercises that involved both floor and standing exercises for core, proximal joint and knee stability;
- Continued yoga two to three times per week.

Evaluation
The patient was reassessed and the programme modified and progressed on a regular basis over a 10-month period.

Ten months after commencement of the programme the patient was reassessed and she reported a marked subjective improvement in general health, fitness, energy levels, sense of wellbeing, strength and coordination. She had experienced reduced frequency and duration of 'flare-ups', less knee pain and improved functional capacity, being able to walk on flat ground without pain and exacerbation of symptoms for over 4 hours. Reassessment showed improved posture, standing balance, proprioception and dynamic trunk stability.

Comment
This highly motivated and committed patient achieved good results with a progressive rehabilitation programme and is expected to achieve her personal fitness goals over the next 6–12 months.

The long-term aim of hill climbing remains a goal to be achieved. Specific lower limb functional muscular training is now required. This will include a graduated aerobic walking and stepping programme in association with specific gluteal, quadriceps and calf conditioning exercises.

CONCLUSION

Designing rehabilitation and fitness programmes for individuals with generalized hypermobility and JHS is a multifactorial challenge. Progress is often hampered by setbacks of reinjury or exacerbation, and patience on the part of both physiotherapist and patient is necessary. However, where there is commitment from both physiotherapist and patient and the most suitable mode and level of paced exercise is prescribed, results can be very rewarding and patients can go on to manage the condition effectively.

Further research into the neuromusculoskeletal, biomechanical and physiological effects of exercise and sport in the hypermobile population is required to assist the further establishment of rehabilitation and management guidelines.

REFERENCES

Acasuso-Diaz, M. and Collantes-Estevez, E. (1998) Joint hypermobility in patients with fibromyalgia. *Arthritis Care Research*, **33**, 39–42.

Akeson, W.H., Amiel, D. and Woo, S. (1980) Immobility effects of synovial joints: the pathomechanics of joint contracture. *Biorheology*, **17**, 95–110.

Ali, H.M. (2001a) Fibromyalgia (case study). *Physiotherapy*, **87**, 140–5.

Ali, M. (2001b) *The Integrated Health Bible*, pp. 158–169.Vermillion.

American College of Sports Medicine (ACSM) (1980) *Guidelines for Graded Exercise Testing and Exercise Prescription*, 2nd edn. Philadelphia: Lea & Febiger.

American College of Sports Medicine (ACSM) (1988) *Resource Manual for Guidelines for Graded Exercise Testing and Exercise Prescription*. Philadelphia: Lea & Febiger.

Beighton, P.H., Grahame, R. and Bird, H. (1989) *Hypermobility of Joints*, 2nd edn. Springer-Verlag.

Bird, S.R., Smith, A., James, K. et al. (1998) Exercise and physical activity: an overview of the benefits. *Exercise Benefits and Prescription*, **1**, 1–15. Stanley Thornes.

Booth, F.W. (1987) Physiological and biochemical effect of immobilization on muscle. *Clinical Orthopedics and Related Research*, **219**, 15–20.

Booth, F.W. and Kelso, J.R. (1973) Effects of hind limb immobilization on contractile and histochemical properties of skeletal muscle. *Pflugers Archiv*, **342**, 231–8.

Burdeaux, B.D. and Hutchinson, W.J. (1953) Etiology of traumatic osteoporosis. *American Journal of Bone and Joint Surgery*, **35**, 479–88.

Butler, D.S. (1991) *Mobilisation of the Nervous System*. Churchill Livingstone.

Cabaud, H.E., Chatty, A. and Gildengorin, V. (1980) Exercise effects on the strength of the rat anterior cruciate ligament. *American Journal of Sports Medicine*, **8**, 79–86.

Carrière, B. (1998) *The Swiss Ball*. Springer-Verlag.

Cherpel, A. and Marks, R. (1999) The benign joint hypermobility syndrome. *New Zealand Journal of Physiotherapy*, **27**, 9–22.

Child, A.H. (1986) Joint hypermobility syndrome: inherited disorder of collagen synthesis. *Journal of Rheumatology*, **113**, 239–43.

Cooper, R.R. (1972) Alternatives during immobilization and regeneration of skeletal muscle in cats. *American Journal of Bone and Joint Surgery*, **54**, 919–53.

Davis, B.C. and Harrison, A.D. (1988) *Hydrotherapy in Practice*. Churchill Livingstone.

Decoster, L., Vailas, J.C., Lindsay, R.H. and Williams, G.R. (1979) Prevalence and features of joint hypermobility among adolescent athletes. *Archives of Pediatric and Adolescent Medicine*, **151**, 989–92.

Egger, G., Champion, N. and Bolton, A. (1998) *The Fitness Leaders Handbook*, 4th edn. Kangaroo Press.

Ekstrand, J. and Gillquist, J. (1983) Soccer injuries and their mechanisms. A prospective study. *Medicine Science Sports Exercise*, **15**, 267–70.

Engles, M. (1994) Tissue response. In *Orthopaedic Physical Medicine* (R. Donatelli and M. Wooden, eds). Churchill Livingstone.

Francis, H., March, L., Terenty, T. and Webb, J. (1987) Benign joint hypermobility with neuropathy: documentation and mechanism of tarsal tunnel syndrome. *Journal of Rheumatology*, **14**, 577–81.

Fuller, C.S. (1998) Aquatic rehabilitation. In *Physical Rehabilitation of the Injured Athlete*, 2nd edn. (J.R. Anderson, G.L. Harrelson and K.E. Wilkes, eds). WB Saunders.

Gazit, Y., Nahir, A.M., Grahame, R. and Jacob, G. (2003) Dysautonomia in the joint hypermobility syndrome. *American Journal of Medicine*, **115**, 33–40.

Gedalia, A. and Brewer, E.J. (1993) Joint hypermobility in paediatric practice: a review. *Journal of Rheumatology*, **20**, 371–4.

Goldman, J.A. (1991) Hypermobility and deconditioning: important links to fibromyalgia/fibrositis. *Southern Medical Journal*, **84**, 1192–6.

Grahame, R. (1971) Joint hypermobility, clinical aspects. *Proceedings of the Royal Society of Medicine*, **64**, 32–4.

Grahame, R. (2000a) Pain, distress and joint hyperlaxity. *Joint Bone Spine*, **6**, 64–70.

Grahame, R. (2000b) Not a circus act. Review. *International Journal of Clinical Practice*, **54**, 314–15.

Grahame, R. and Jenkins, J.M. (1972) Joint hypermobility: asset or liability. *Annals of the Rheumatic Diseases*, **31**, 109–11.

Grahame, R., Hunt, J.N., Kitchen, S. and Gabel, A. (1978) The diuretic, natriuretic and kaluretic effects of water immersion. *Quarterly Journal of Medicine*, **45**, 579.

Grahame, R., Edwards, J.C., Pitcher, D. et al. (1981) A clinical and echographic study of patients with the hypermobility syndrome. *Annals of the Rheumatic Diseases*, **49**, 190–200.

Grana, W.A. and Moretz, J.A. (1985) Ligament laxity in secondary school athletes. *Journal of the American Medical Association*, **240**, 1975–6.

Guskiewicz, K.M. and Perrin, D.H. (1996) Research and clinical applications of assessing balance. *Journal of Sports Rehabilitation*, **5**, 45–63.

Hall, M.G., Ferrell, W.R., Sturrock, R.D., et al. (1995) The effect of the hypermobility syndrome on knee joint proprioception. *British Journal of Rheumatology*, **34**, 121–5.

Hardt, A.B. (1972) Early metabolic responses of bone to immobilization. *American Journal of Bone and Joint Surgery*, **54**, 119–24.

Harrelson, G.L. (1998) Physiological factors of rehabilitation. In: *Physical Rehabilitation of the Injured Athlete*, 2nd edn. (R.J. Andrews et al. eds), pp. 13–37. WB Saunders.

Harrelson, G.L. and Leaver-Dunn, D. (1998) Introduction to rehabilitation. In: *Physical Rehabilitation of the Injured Athlete*, 2nd edn. (R.J. Andrews et al. eds), pp. 175–217. WB Saunders.

Hides, J., Stokes, M., Saide, M. et al. (1994) Evidence of lumbar multifidus muscle wasting ipsilateral to symptoms in patients with acute/subacute low back pain. *Spine*, **19**, 165–70.

Hinton, R.Y. (1986) Case study: rehabilitation of multiple joint instability associated with Ehlers–Danlos syndrome. *Journal of Orthopaedic and Sports Physical Therapy*, **84**, 193–8.

Hodges, P. and Richardson, C. (1996) Inefficient muscular stabilization of the lumbar spine associated with low back pain: a motor control evaluation of transversus abdominis. *Physiotherapy Research International*, **1**, 30–40.

Hurley, R. and Turner, C. (1991) Neurology and aquatic therapy. *Clinical Management*, **11**, 26–29.

Irwin, S. (1994) Exercise treatment for the rehabilitated patient: cardiopulmonary and peripheral responses. In: *Orthopaedic Physical Therapy*, 2nd edn. (R. Donatelli and M.J. Wooden, eds), pp. 33–41. Churchill Livingstone.

Jull, G. (2001) A management programme for cervicogenic headache and neck pain patients. In: *Cervical Spine and Whiplash Research Unit, Department of Physiotherapy. The University of Queensland Australia*. A teaching publication produced by University of Queensland.

Keller, C.S., Noyes, F.R. and Buncher, C.R. (1987) The medical aspects of soccer injury epidemiology. *American Journal of Sports Medicine*, **15**, 230–7.

Kendall, F.P., McCreary, E.K. and Provance, P.G. (1983) *Muscles: Testing and Function*, 3rd edn. Williams & Wilkins, Maryland.

Kennedy, J.C., Alexander, I.J. and Hayes, K.C. (1982) Nerve supply of the human knee and its functional importance. *American Journal of Sports Medicine*, **10**, 329–35.

Kerr, A., Macmillan, C.E., Uttley, W. and Luqmani, R.A. (2000) Physiotherapy for children with hypermobility syndrome. *Physiotherapy*, **86**, 313–16.

Kirkby, R.L., Simms, C., Symington, V.J. et al. (1981) Flexibility and musculoskeletal symptomatology in female gymnasts and age-matched controls. *American Journal of Sports Medicine*, **9**, 160–4.

Klemp, P. and Learmouth, I.D. (1984) Hypermobility and injuries in a professional ballet company. *British Journal of Sport Medicine*, **18**, 143–8.

Lamb, D.R. (1984) *Physiology of Exercise*. Collier Macmillan, London.

Landry, M. and Fleisch, H. (1964) The influence of immobilization on bone formation as evaluated by osseous incorporation of tetracyclines. *British Journal of Bone and Joint Surgery*, **46**, 764–71.

Laros, G.S., Tipton, C. and Cooper, R.R. (1971) Influence of physical activity on ligament insertions in the knees of dogs. *American Journal of Bone and Joint Surgery*, **53**, 275–86.

Lephart, S. (1994) Re-establishing proprioception, kinaesthesia, joint position sense and neuromuscular control in rehabilitation. In: *Rehabilitation Techniques in Sports Medicine* (W.E. Prentice, ed.). St. Louis, C.V. Mosby.

Lephart, S.M., Perrin, D.H. and Fu, F.H. (1992) Proprioception following anterior cruciate reconstruction. *Journal of Sports Rehabilitation*, **1**, 188–96.

Lysens R.J., Ostyn, M.S., Auweele, Y.V. et al. (1989) The accident prone and overuse prone profiles of the young athlete. *American Journal of Sports Medicine*, **17**, 612–19.

MacDougall, J.D., Ward, G.R., Sale, D.G. et al. (1977) Effects of strength training and immobilization on human muscle fibres. *European Journal of Applied Physiology*, **43**, 700–3.

Macsween, A., Brydson, G., Creed, G. and Capell, H.A. (2001) A preliminary validation of the 10-metre incremental shuttle walk test as a measure of aerobic capacity in women with rheumatoid arthritis. *Physiotherapy*, **87**, 38–44.

Mallik, A.K., Ferrell, W.R., McDonald, A.G. and Sturrock, R.D. (1994) Impaired proprioceptive acuity at the proximal interphalangeal joint in patients with the hypermobility syndrome. *British Journal of Rheumatology*, **33**, 631–7.

Melzack, R. (1987) The short McGill Pain Questionnaire. *Pain*, **30**, 191–7.

Morgan, A.W., Peerson, S.B., Bird, H.A. (1996) Respiratory symptoms in Ehlers–Danlos syndrome and the benign joint hypermobility syndrome. *Arthritis and Rheumatism* **39**(9) S136 (Abstract).

Nicolas, J.A. (1970) Injuries to knee ligaments. Relationship to looseness and tightness in football players. *Journal of the American Medical Association*, **212**, 2236–9.

Noyes, F.R., Mangine, R.E. and Barber, S. (1974) Biomechanics of ligament failure. II. An analysis of immobilization, exercise and reconditioning effects in primates. *American Journal of Bone and Joint Surgery*, **56**, 1406–18.

O'Sullivan, P., Twomey, L. and Allison, G. (1997) Dynamic stabilization of the lumbar spine. *Critical Reviews in Physical Rehabilitation Medicine*, **9**, 315.

Panjabi, M.M. (1992) The stabilizing system of the spine. Function, dysfunction, adaptation and enhancement. *Journal of Spinal Disorders*, **5**, 383–9.

Petajan J.H., Gappmaier, E, White, A.T. et al. (1996) Impact of aerobic training on fitness and quality of life in multiple sclerosis. *Annals of Neurology*, **39**, 432–41.

Rasch, P.J. and Burke, R.K. (1977) *Kinesiology and Applied Anatomy*, 6th edn. pp. 417–44. Lea & Febiger.

Rifenberick, D.H. and Max, S.R. (1974) Substrate utilization by disused rat skeletal muscles. *American Journal of Physiology*, **226**, 295–7.

Sahrmann, S. (2002) *Diagnosis and Treatment of Movement Impairment Syndromes*. Mosby.

Schultz, R.A., Miller, D.C. and Kerr, C.S. (1984) Mechanoreceptors in human cruciate ligament: a histological study. *American Journal of Bone and Joint Surgery*, **69**, 1072–6.

Shoen, R.P., Kirsner, A.B., Farber, S.J. and Finkel, R.I. (1982) The hypermobility syndrome. *Postgraduate Medicine*, **71**, 199–208.

Skinner, H.B., Wyatt, M.P. and Hudgdon, J.A. (1986) Effect of fatigue on joint position of the knee. *Journal of Orthopedic Research*, **4**, 112–18.

Skinner, A.T. and Thomson, A.M. (1993) *Duffield's Exercise in Water*, 3rd edn, pp. 44 and 141–3. London: Baillière Tindall.

Steinberg, F.U. (1980) *The Immobilized Patient: Functional Pathology and Management*. Millen Press, New York.

Steiner, M.E. (1987) Hypermobility and knee injuries. *Physician and Sports Medicine*, **15**, 159–65.

Tipton, C.M., James, S.L., Mergner, W. et al. (1970) Influence of exercise on strength of medial collateral knee ligaments of dogs. *American Journal of Physiology*, **218**, 894–902.

Vincenzo, B. (1995) Considerations in injury prevention. In: *Sports Physiotherapy* (M. Zaluagu, ed.). Churchill Livingstone.

Vleeming, A., Snijders, C.J., Stoeckart, R. et al. (1995) The posterior layer of the thoracolumbar fascia: its function in load transfer from spine to legs. *Spine* **20**, 753–8.

Willis, W.D. and Grossman, R.G. (1981) *Medical Neurobiology*, 3rd edn. St. Louis: Mosby.

Witzmann, F.A., Kim, D.H. and Fitts, R.H. (1982) Recovery time course in recovery function of fast and slow skeletal muscle after hindlimb immobilization. *Journal of Applied Physiology*, **52**, 677–82.

Wolfe, F., Smythe, H.A., Younus, M.B. et al. (1990) The American College of Rheumatology 1990 criteria for classification of fibromyalgia. *Arthritis and Rheumatism*, **33**, 160–72.

Woo, SL-Y, Gomez, M.A., Young-Kyun, W. et al. (1982) Mechanical properties of tendons and ligaments II: the relationship of immobilization and exercise on tissue remodelling. *Biorheology*, **19**, 397.

Worsford, C. and Simpson, J.M. (2001) Standardisation of a three-metre walking test for the elderly. *Physiotherapy*, **87**, 25–132.

Zarins, B. (1982) Soft tissue injury and repair: biomechanical aspects. *International Journal of Sports Medicine*, **3**, 19–25.

9

Joint hypermobility and work-related musculoskeletal disorders (WRMSD)

Jean Mangharam

Aims

1. To provide the reader with background information about WRMSD, including the definition, associated risk factors, proposed pathogeneses, and the associated biological responses and pathology
2. To explore the potential impact of having hypermobile joints and lax tissue on the development of WRMSD
3. To discuss pertinent ergonomic principles and propose suitable applications.

DEFINITION OF WORK-RELATED MUSCULOSKELETAL DISORDERS (WRMSD)

The prevalence of musculoskeletal disorders (primarily of the neck, upper limb and back) among the workforce of European Union Member States and the United States of America is high and continues to be a major reason for illness and financial burden in the workplace (Violante et al. 2000, European Agency for Safety and Health at Work (EASHW) 1999, Kumar 2001). There is growing worldwide concern about the prevalence of musculoskeletal disorders in the workplace. International meetings and workshops such as the one carried out in April 1998 by the World Health Organization in Sweden, and several large-scale projects to investigate the problem, have been commissioned by national and international bodies. Three such investigations and reviews include:

- **NIOSH (1997)** The National Institute for Occupational Safety and Health (USA) carried out an extensive critical review of epidemiological evidence for work-related musculoskeletal disorders for the neck, upper extremity and low back. The review identified a number of specific physical exposures strongly associated with specific WRMSD, especially when exposures were intense, prolonged, and particularly when workers were exposed to several risk factors.

- **European Agency for Safety and Health at Work (EASHW) (1999)** The European Agency for Safety and Health at Work requested the Robbens Institute, University of Surrey, to describe and assess findings of relevant research related to work-related upper limb disorders (WRULD). The review was detailed and systematic in its presentation of the nature of the problem, and proposed models of pathogenesis, biological responses and strategies for prevention.

- **National Research Council (1999)** The National Institutes of Health (NIH) in the USA requested that the National Academy of Sciences and National Research Council convene a panel of experts to carefully examine questions raised by Congress concerning occupational musculoskeletal disorders. Comprehensive information related to tissue mechanics, biological responses and proposed theories about the interaction between workplace extrinsic and individual intrinsic factors were presented.

'Work-related musculoskeletal disorders' (WRMSD) is an umbrella term used to describe musculoskeletal disorders which have been associated with the work of the affected person. The term 'work-related upper limb disorders' (WRULD) refers particularly to work-related musculoskeletal disorders of the neck and upper limb. Several terms have been used to describe WRULD, including repetitive strain injury (RSI in Australia and the UK), occupational overuse syndrome (OOS in Australia), cumulative trauma disorders (CTD in USA), occupational cervicobrachial disorder (OCBD in Japan, Switzerland and Sweden), tension headache and occupational disorder (in Finland) and Occupational Complaint Number 2101 (in the former Federal Republic of Germany) (Ireland 1995).

The term WRMSD does not suggest or imply aetiology, nor specify a risk factor or anatomical region affected. It suggests that the disorder is musculoskeletal in nature and is related to the occupation of those affected. The primary reason for the controversy surrounding the terminology and classification of WRMSD is its complex multifactorial aetiology, progression and prognosis (NIOSH 1997, Mayer et al. 2000). The World Health Organization clarified this by stating that 'Work-related diseases may be partially caused by adverse working conditions. They may be aggravated, accelerated or exacerbated by workplace exposures and they may impair working capacity. Personal characteristics and other environmental and sociocultural factors usually play a role as risk factors in work-related diseases; which may often be more common than occupational disease' (WHO 1985, Identification and Control of Work Related Diseases. Technical Report No. 174. General: World Health Organization, cited in National Research Council and Institute of Medicine 2001).

RISK FACTORS ASSOCIATED WITH WRMSD

Multifactorial

NIOSH (1997) found that the epidemiological studies investigating the role of physical factors, work organizational and psychosocial factors in the development of WRMSD for the neck, shoulder, elbow, hand and back were not guided by an established and consistent definition of WRMSD. The presentation of WRMSD may have been based on clinical pathology, the presence of symptoms, objective pathological processes and/or work disability (e.g. days away from work). Of the studies reviewed, the most common health outcome was the occurrence of pain.

NIOSH (1997) and European Agency for Safety and Health at Work (1999) have both stated that the lack of standardized criteria for defining WRMSD makes investigation and comparison between studies difficult. NIOSH (1997) points out that it would be useful to have a concise pathophysiological definition and corresponding objective clinical test for each WRMSD, to translate the degree of tissue damage or dysfunction into an estimate of current or future disability and prognosis. However, clinically defined WRMSD often have no clearly delineated pathophysiological mechanisms for pathological processes.

Reviews of studies have shown that the physical risk factors that have been associated with WRMSD include repetitive movement, forceful movements, heavy physical work, awkward postures, static postures, contact stress (local mechanical pressure or high-impact external forces), hand-tool vibration, whole body vibration and cool temperatures (NIOSH 1997, European Agency for Safety and Health at Work 1999, National Research Council 1999).

NIOSH (1997) summarized the causal relationship between physical work factors and WRMSD (Table 9.1). The studies reviewed displayed strong evidence of a causal relationship between posture as a risk factor on neck/shoulder disorders; a combination of risk factors (repetition, force and posture) on elbow disorders; a combination of physical risk factors (repetition, force, posture and vibration) on carpal tunnel syndrome; a combination of physical risk factors (repetition, force and posture) on hand/wrist tendonitis, vibration on hand-arm vibration syndrome; and lifting/forceful movements and whole body vibration on

Table 9.1 Evidence for causal relationship between physical work and WRMSD (NIOSH 1997)

Body part Risk factor	Strong evidence	Evidence	Insufficient evidence	Evidence of no effect
Neck and neck/shoulder				
Repetition		✔		
Force		✔		
Posture	✔			
Vibration			✔	
Shoulder				
Posture		✔		
Force			✔	
Repetition		✔		
Vibration			✔	
Elbow				
Repetition			✔	
Force		✔		
Posture			✔	
Combination	✔			
Hand/wrist – carpal tunnel syndrome				
Repetition		✔		
Force		✔		
Posture			✔	
Vibration		✔		
Combination	✔			
Hand/wrist – tendonitis				
Repetition		✔		
Force		✔		
Posture		✔		
Combination	✔			
Hand–arm vibration syndrome				
Vibration	✔			
Back				
Lifting/ forceful movements	✔			
Awkward posture		✔		
Heavy physical work		✔		
Whole body vibration	✔			
Static work posture			✔	

back disorders. There was insufficient evidence of a causal relationship between vibration and neck/shoulder disorders; force and vibration on shoulder disorders; repetition and posture on elbow disorders; posture on carpal tunnel syndrome; and static work postures on back disorders. It was pointed out that high-risk jobs would typically be composed of tasks that expose the worker to one or more risk factors.

MODELS FOR THE PATHOGENESIS OF WRMSD

Several conceptual models have been designed to explain how multiple factors may interact to increase the propensity of an individual to develop a work-related musculoskeletal disorder.

A dose–response model for neck and upper limb disorders was developed by researchers from Denmark, Finland, Sweden, England and the United States (Armstrong et al. 1993). The model described four domains: exposure, dose, capacity and response. These factors interact within a model which considers the intrinsic and extrinsic influencing factors. This model emphasizes the cumulative nature of work-related neck and upper limb disorders.

A model developed by the National Research Council (1999) shows how environmental work factors and the individual's personal factors can have an impact on the physiological pathways, progression and outcome of a WRMSD. The model shows how individual factors and external factors, including external loads, organizational factors and social context, can have an influence on the biomechanical loading (internal loading and physiological responses), internal tolerances (mechanical strain and subsequent fatigue) and outcomes (pain/discomfort and subsequent impairment/disability). Arrows between the workplace factors and the person (Fig. 9.1) indicate the various research disciplines (epidemiology, biomechanics, physiology etc.) that have attempted to explain the relationship.

The model incorporates the role of various factors associated with WRMSD, including work procedures, equipment, environment, organizational factors, individual physical and psychological factors, non-work related activities and social factors. The central physiological pathway shows the biomechanical relationship between load and the biological response of tissue. Loads of various magnitudes can change the form of tissues throughout the day (e.g. changes secondary to fatigue and work pattern or style). The biomechanical loading can lead to symptomatic and asymptomatic responses. If the load exceeds a mechanical tolerance, tissue damage or reactions will occur. The feedback mechanisms (e.g. pain) can influence the biomechanical loading

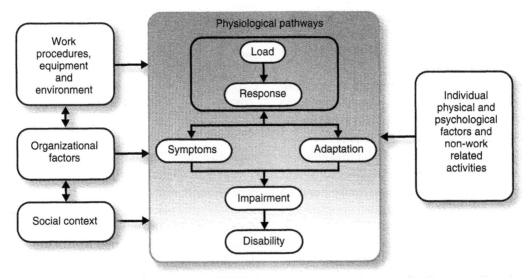

Figure 9.1 Conceptual framework of physiological pathways and factors that potentially contribute to musculoskeletal disorders from National Research Council 1999, with permission from the National Academy of Sciences

and load–response relationship. Adaptation may increase the tolerance for greater biomechanical loading, or allow tissues to sustain a greater load until tissue tolerance is exceeded. The symptom and adaptation outcome may subsequently interact with each other. Functional impairment may result from the responses, symptoms and adaptations. Disability may ensue if the resultant impairment is severe. Similarly, and sometimes concurrently with physical loading, undesirable organizational factors and the social context, if sufficiently intense, can influence the way in which the individual will respond and progress with problems. Individual physical and psychological factors and non-work related activities may also have an influence on the physiological pathways.

Repetitive movement

Definition

Repetitive movement usually refers to the execution of cyclical patterns of movement without regular pauses or breaks between the cycles. These cyclical movement patterns are usually executed to complete subtasks within a task, and a job would usually be composed of a variety of tasks. The level of risk imposed by repetitive movement will depend on the frequency of the cycle, the force required during the movement, the duration of the cyclical movement, the frequency and duration of breaks within and between subtasks, and the total cumulative exposure period. Often, the upper limbs, especially the smaller joints (e.g. fingers and wrists), are dynamic during repetitive movement, as these tasks usually require high manual dexterity (e.g. typing or playing a musical instrument). During these tasks, central and core muscles contract to stabilize the skeletal system while peripheral musculature carries out repetitive contraction and relaxation (e.g. keyboard interaction requires repetitive finger flexion/extension/abduction/adduction while the wrist, elbow, shoulder and shoulder girdle remain static).

Repetitive movement: biological responses and pathology

It has been found that repeated loading of tendons, especially if the load is tensile and in a transverse direction (e.g. gripping, passing bony structures or adjacent tissue, in awkward postures or end of range), increases the risk of an injury (Armstrong et al. 1984, Goldstein et al. 1987). The collagen fibres may separate from one another following repetitive activity, resulting in swelling and pain (Chaffin and Andersen 1991). The swelling may change the coefficient of friction between the tendon and the sheath, leading to irritation of the tissues as the tendon glides repetitively within its sheath. A tendonitis or tenosynovitis may result. Histological changes have been found following tendon loading (Backman et al. 1990).

Repetitive movement: vulnerability of the hypermobile individual

Joint hypermobility syndrome (JHS) patients have been thought to be susceptible to tendonitis of the upper and lower limbs. The explanation may be that there is a variation in the properties of their tendon collagen. Both deficiencies in collagen production and deficiencies in collagen turnover have now been recognized in different variants of Ehlers–Danlos syndrome (EDS) (Beighton et al. 1998, Miller and Gay 1987). Garcia-Cruz et al. (1998) found defective connective tissue in familial articular hypermobility syndrome. Biochemical (collagen types) and morphological variations were found (general disorganization of dermal components, showing a loose collagen network characterized by thick bundles).

Despite the above findings, Larsson et al. (1993) suggests that hypermobility may be an asset to musicians, who require repetitive movement of their joints. Results showed that musculoskeletal symptoms associated with practice and performance may be due to lack of hypermobility of some joints involved in intensive repetitive movement. Subjects who played instruments requiring much more repetitive motion had symptoms that affected their joints less often if the joints involved were hypermobile than if they were not. Larsson et al. (1995) reinforced their findings in industrial workers, when they showed that the individual with a hypermobile spine was less susceptible to back pain, in jobs requiring changing body postures.

Force

Definition

Force may be a risk factor in situations when the force required to carry out a task (one-off or cumulative) exceeds that which can be created (active) or withstood (passive) by the individual's musculoskeletal system. Excessive stress or strain can result from a single forceful mechanical event (e.g. lifting, catching), from an interaction with the environment (e.g. a fall), or from accumulated strain associated with loading of a structure. Probably – and more commonly – excessive tissue strain can be caused by a combination of a single high-force event superimposed on weak structures secondary to a history of repetitive loading (Ashton-Miller 1999). Force can be defined as external or internal, imposed either externally as a load, or internally created by a motor response or passive tensile stretch of connective tissue.

Force: biological responses and pathology

Muscle injury The sarcomeres of muscles may be damaged morphologically at focal points secondary to mechanical disruption during contraction-induced injuries. The inflammatory response may further damage the muscle units. Striated muscle appears to be at higher risk of being damaged during activation and being forcibly stretched, rather than during the isometric phase of muscular contraction. The stretch may be self-initiated or secondary to external loading (Ashton-Miller 1999). Edwards (1988) hypothesized that eccentric contractions have a high potential for muscle damage.

Passive tensile structures Collagen provides the tensile strength in dense regular connective tissue. Collagen is an extremely active substance that is sensitive to loading history. Fluctuating loading usually promotes collagen turnover, whereas static loading may lead to collagen atrophy. The turnover in avascular structures such as intervertebral discs takes much longer, and the various types of collagen have different turnover rates (Ashton-Miller 1999).

Joint surface Radwin and Lavender (1999) discussed the findings of bone response to internal tissue loading. Several authors have reported that osteoarthritis in the hip and knees is more prevalent in individuals employed in occupations that experience greater loading of the lower extremity.

Intervertebral disc Researchers have found that prolapsed discs occur more frequently in the forward flexed position (Adams and Hutton 1982). In flexion, the anterior portion undergoes compression and the posterior portion of the annulus fibrosis is under tensile stretch. The disc, especially the vertebral endplate, is particularly susceptible to repetitive loading and large compressive forces in the forward flexed position (Radwin and Lavender 1999).

Force: vulnerability of the hypermobile individual

For the hypermobile individual, it appears that several structures may be vulnerable when high forces are imposed. Muscle strain has not particularly been presented as an issue for the hypermobile individual. However, passive tensile structures, bone structures and joint surfaces have been presented as being vulnerable for the hypermobile individual when placed under stress.

Magnusson et al. (2001) showed that the passive properties of the hamstring muscle tendon unit of JHS patients are similar to those of controls. However, their results suggest that JHS patients have a greater subjective tolerance to passive stretch, displaying greater maximal stretch angle (stretch sensation without pain) and corresponding peak moment.

Nijs et al. (2000) found that spinal and femoral bone densities (volumetric total and cortical bone at the radius) were lower in hypermobile individuals, after correction for body mass index. Comparisons were made between 25 female (Caucasian) hypermobile individuals aged between 19 and 57 years, and a corresponding age-matched reference population. In contrast, an earlier study by Mishra et al. (1996) found that although 31% of 58 patients with joint hypermobility syndrome had significant arthralgia, there was no significant reduction in bone mineral density.

Proprioception is critical for the maintenance of joint stability. Studies have demonstrated that proprioception is less accurate in patients with hypermobility syndrome (Hall et al. 1995). Pathways between proprioceptive inaccuracy, knee osteoarthritis and related knee disorders have been suggested (Sharma 1999, Sharma and Pai 1997).

The vertebral column is stabilized by intersegmental muscles (e.g. multifidus, rotares, interspinales and intertransversarii) (Oliver and Middleditch, 2000). Whereas spinal stability tends to occur at the segmental level, the more superficial longitudinal muscles counterbalance external loads and achieve movement more successfully. Proprioception at the segmental level would therefore be especially beneficial to reduce the risk of injury of the facet joints and intervertebral discs. Because of proprioception limitations, the hypermobile individual has been thought to be at greater risk of spinal injury. Howes and Isdale (1971) stated that the 'loose back' syndrome is accepted as being more common than originally thought.

Despite findings from the above studies, Larsson et al. (1995) showed that there were no significant effects of tasks involving heavy lifting on hypermobile versus non-hypermobile individuals. However, the number of industrial workers whose primary tasks involved heavy lifting in the study was limited (12 females and 24 males).

Beighton et al. (1999) pointed out that throughout the literature it is widely thought that premature osteoarthritis may be a direct consequence of hypermobility. However, final proof may only follow a large and perspective long-term study (Beighton et al. 1998).

Awkward posture

Definition

Awkward posture, as a risk factor, usually refers to working in a joint range that is not in neutral and which is often not optimal for muscular force generation. Awkward postures may result from an individual engaging in poor or suboptimal work practices and postures, or working with poor tool design, furniture design, equipment design and/or physical man–machine interfaces.

Awkward postures: biological responses and pathology

Awkward postures often require muscles to exert a force in a range which is not optimal for force generation (either in shortened or lengthened position), potentially leading to strain. Awkward postures may also place adverse forces on joint surfaces which are not coupled with congruence, or compressive and stretching forces on various components of the musculoskeletal system, including muscles, discs, tendons, joint capsules, ligaments, connective tissue and nerve tissue. Should the awkward postures be repeated or sustained during static work, impairments of various components of the musculoskeletal system and their interaction may be affected. Lengths and the extensibility of various components of the musculoskeletal system may be altered and movement impairment may result (Sahrmann 2002). Hypertrophy or shortening of certain muscles and atrophy and lengthening of others may in the long term lead to a muscular imbalance, especially if the postural muscles that provide stability close to the joints are not adequately recruited regularly, for maintenance of neutral posturing.

It has been shown that awkward posture of a single joint (shoulder flexion alone) can lead to increased discomfort, muscular fatigue (detected by EMG changes) and reduced performance (Straker et al. 1997).

Awkward postures: vulnerability of the hypermobile individual

It is expected that the hypermobile individual will be especially vulnerable to working in awkward postures for sustained periods. Such individuals may be particularly vulnerable to muscular imbalances, as the deep core muscles fail to stabilize joints owing to poor proprioception during prolonged awkward static postures. Repetitive awkward postures may not pose as great a risk at the hypermobile joints, because of the greater extensibility of these joints. Silverman et al. (1975) demonstrated that a clinically hypermobile individual has greater extensibility of the fifth right metacarpophalangeal joint by displaying the joint angle response to increasing loads. The load versus joint angle curves showed that less load was required to extend the joint to similar angles as in controls, and the hypermobile individual showed greater extensibility of that joint. The authors also showed that the extensibility of joints is inversely correlated with age. However, should damage occur, the alterations in collagen turnover and defects in connective tissue, as seen in Ehlers–Danlos syndrome (Miller and Gay 1987) may leave the individual at risk of experiencing greater musculoskeletal problems, especially with increased age.

Static postures

Definition

During prolonged static postures low-level muscular contraction is required to maintain the stability of a body segment. It has been suggested that muscular fatigue, tissue compression and alteration in tissue extensibility may result in and lead to movement impairment and muscular imbalances.

Static postures: biological responses and pathology

Sustained postural muscle activity may lead to muscle fatigue. Research has shown that muscle fatigue does affect proprioceptive acuity. Because proprioception is known to be important for motor control, it has been hypothesized that alteration in inhibition can increase coactivation, inefficient muscle use and the workload of the muscle affected (Ashton-Miller 1999).

It has been suggested that at low-level contraction adjacent blood vessels and nerves are compressed for prolonged periods, limiting blood flow and nerve conduction to the periphery (Grandjean 1982). Hagberg and Hagberg (1989) reported that at 30° of shoulder abduction, the perfusion of the supraspinatus muscle may decrease as the intramuscular pressure increases with static contraction of the muscle. Decreased blood flow in the supraspinatus may cause degeneration of the tendon and rotator cuff tendonitis.

Veiersted et al. (1993) found that myalgia may result at low prolonged contraction levels. Jonsson (1982) hypothesized that myalgia was secondary to ischaemia due to high static load, with resultant occlusion or impedance of circulation. Hägg (1998, cited in EASHW 1999) hypothesized that myalgia may be associated with a specific pattern of muscle recruitment, where selected muscle fibres and motor units become vulnerable. There is evidence of variance between the characteristics of the fibres in those exposed to high repetitive and static workloads compared to those who have not been exposed to these factors. The irregularities observed appear to be related to the fibre mitochondria. Hägg (1998) suggests that mitochondrial disturbances in type 1 (recruited for static load exertion) muscle fibres in the upper trapezius muscle follow exposure to static and repetitive workload. Hägg suggests that these types of muscle abnormalities may be a necessary but not sufficient condition for pain perception.

The physiological mechanism underlying muscle fibre abnormalities in the upper trapezius muscle following static loads and complaints of myalgia are only partially understood (Hägg 1998). This is due partly to methodological difficulties in taking muscle fibre from human subjects.

Static postures: vulnerability of the hypermobile individual

Larsson et al. (1993) found that the daily problems caused by hypermobility in musicians were not related to the total number of hypermobile joints in a subject but rather to the use of certain joints when playing particular instruments. The percentage of subjects with hypermobile knees who reported symptoms was significantly higher ($P < 0.001$) than the corresponding percentage among the subjects without such hypermobility. The proportion of subjects with hypermobility of the spine who had symptoms involving the back was significantly higher than the proportion of those who did not have hypermobility. The authors felt that hypermobility of the spine, and to some extent of the knees, can be a liability during long periods of practice and performance in the erect posture, as an overuse syndrome (i.e. pain in muscles involved in support function) may be presenting. Larsson et al. (1995) found similar results when he analysed the effects of task types on industrial workers. The authors found that workers with hypermobility experienced more back pain with sitting or standing jobs than workers without hypermobility. The corresponding numbers with back pain for jobs with changing postures were greater for those without hypermobility. The authors once again concluded that hypermobility is an asset if the work requires changes of body posture, but a liability for those requiring static joints.

Whole body vibration (WBV)

Definition

Whole body vibration refers to mechanical energy oscillations which are transferred to the body as a whole. The motion is usually measured in the 'x' (front to back), 'y' (side to side) and 'z' (up and down) directions. Once the direction of vibration is defined the frequency and amplitude must also be specified. The exposure to whole body vibration usually takes place through a supporting seat or platform, generally in transportation vehicles (e.g. bus drivers, truck drivers).

Whole body vibration: biological responses and pathology

Bovenzi (2000) states that studies show that there is an excess risk of sciatic pain and lumbar disc disorders, including herniated disc, in the WBV-exposed occupational groups compared to control groups. Mechanical overload and excessive muscular fatigue has been shown by biodynamic and physiological experiments.

Physical changes and disc herniations have been caused in motion segments by exposure to cyclic and vibration loading. A vehicle driver is thought to also be at further risk when unloading, owing to back muscles that have fatigued following exposure to vibration (Pope et al. 2000).

Whole body vibration: vulnerability of the hypermobile individual

There has been no study found which proposes that the hypermobile individual is more susceptible to problems following exposure to whole body vibration. However, because of the vulnerability of hypermobile individuals to collagen damage and intervertebral disc dysfunction, caution is recommended in exposure to WBV.

Cool temperatures

Cool temperatures: biological responses and pathology

Studies suggest that the physiological demands on muscle and related tissue will be greater for a given task in a cold environment (EASHW 1999).

Increased muscle activity may arise from direct cooling of tissue or postural changes.

Cool temperatures: vulnerability of the hypermobile individual

The hypermobile individual may be more susceptible to cooler environments. Joint hypermobility and bilateral occlusion of the ulnar arteries presenting as Raynaud's phenomenon have been written about (Haberhauer et al. 2000). Beighton et al. (1999) pointed out that alterations in the total volume and weaving of collagen may result from external forces, and that collagen fibres may suffer contractions when the temperature of their surroundings is changed.

Psychosocial issues

Psychosocial issues: biological responses and pathology

Poor job or work organization, particularly lack of sufficient control of the work by the user, under-utilization of skills, high-speed repetitive working or social isolation have been linked with stress in the workplace today. Increased specialization may result in jobs that require repetitive movement and/or static positioning. Such jobs are also usually associated with low job control.

It has been shown that there is an inverse relationship between physical load and job control (MacDonald et al. 2001). MacDonald et al. 2001 found that the correlation between physical and psychosocial stressors was strongest in blue-collar production and low-status office workers, supporting their hypothesis that covariation is more pronounced in groups with greater task specialization. The factors that were especially strongly correlated were low decision latitude and physical loading. Mental demands were usually negative with physical loading. The relationships were weaker in white-collar workers.

It has been shown that psychological stress can increase muscular tension (Waersted and Westgaard 1996, Melin and Lundberg 1997).

Psychosocial issues: vulnerability of the hypermobile individual

It has been pointed out that psychosocial problems may be experienced secondary to pain associated with joint hypermobility (Grahame 2000). Although no specific studies relate work satisfaction and hypermobile individuals, it must be borne in mind that the interaction between unsatisfactory work situations and stresses experienced secondary to pain may leave the hypermobile individual more susceptible and potentiate the risk of problems related to psychosocial issues.

APPLICATION OF ERGONOMIC PRINCIPLES TO REDUCE THE RISK OF WRMSD IN THE HYPERMOBILE INDIVIDUAL

The word 'ergonomics' is Greek in origin and means natural laws (*nomo*) of work (*ergo*). One of the guiding principles of the science is creating a balance between the demands of a task and the capabilities of the individual performing that task (Fig. 9.2).

When the demands of a task, whether physical or mental, are greater than the capability of the individual doing the work in a specific environment, stress (physical or psychological), and consequently strain and injury, may result.

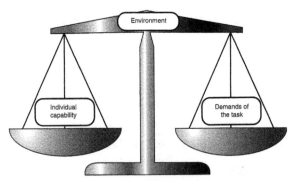

Figure 9.2 A primary ergonomics principle: creating a balance between job task demands and individual capabilities in the work environment

For individuals who have limited physical and psychological capabilities, or for tasks that are highly demanding, the application of ergonomics is especially important. What must be borne in mind is that the balance between individual capability and the demand of the task is also highly influenced by the environment where this balance must take place. For the hypermobile individual physical capacity may be limited relative to certain risk factors of a task, such as high force and static postures, but increased for other factors of a task, such as repetitive movement or extreme joint range requirements.

Ergonomics: the balance

The identification of risks, especially in the context of the essential functions of the job, is the first step in minimizing the risks associated with WRMSD. Once high-risk tasks are identified, specific risk factors can be objectively quantified using currently available tools.

Risk exposure may be reduced by:

- Redesigning a job so that high-risk tasks are eliminated and not required;
- Redesigning the way in which a task is carried out, so that there is less risk;
- Providing or designing equipment, tools and man–machine interfaces to make the task easy to complete;
- Training people or providing them with guiding procedures.

For any organization or individual (including the hypermobile), ergonomic principles may be applied at all three levels of prevention: primary (prevention of onset of injury is a priority), secondary (the goal is to prevent disability and restore function quickly) and tertiary (when physical impairment may already be present, but prevention against further injury or impairment is required to reduce the injury–disability cycle) (Khalil et al. 1999).

Primary prevention

Surveillance: identifying vulnerable joints and tissue

The vulnerability of the hypermobile individual relative to work-related risk factors will depend on what the task and total job requirements are in relation to the individual's grade of hypermobility, past medical history and specificity, and/or the location of hypermobile joints. The ergonomist's awareness of the individual's past medical and current history of hypermobility will provide greater ability to compare and match the individual with the physical and psychological demands of their job. Creating a match between the job and the user is usually attempted by altering the job requirements initially. If the task or environment cannot be modified, guidance regarding the avoidance of high-risk tasks is indicated. For example, a hypermobile individual with a history of lower back pain may choose to work as a cashier. As practitioners, we may expect that individual to be especially vulnerable to prolonged sitting or standing postures. Should they continue working as a cashier without the ability to break away from that position, it is recommended that they alter their posture intermittently between sitting and standing, at an appropriate frequency, to reduce prolonged static positioning.

Currently there is no scientific evidence that validates the use of preassignment medical examinations, job simulation tests or other screening tests as a valid predictor of which employees are likely to develop WRMSD (Hales and Bertsche, 1999). However, a case for the introduction of simple hypermobility screening for those destined to participate in pursuits with a high risk of injury has been made (March and Silman 1993).

Education and training: awareness of risk factors and recommended posture, work practices and manual handling techniques

Understanding the potential problems of joint hypermobility and high tissue laxity relative to potential work-related risk factors is imperative for all parties involved in determining optimal ergonomic settings for the hypermobile individual, including the ergonomist, the individual themselves, and personnel who have an influence on selecting and designating tasks for them. Issues and factors about which it would be important to have an understanding include:

- High-risk work-related factors, including static postures, high loading (force or repetition) on connective tissues, possibly whole body vibration, possible cold environments and possible high-risk psychosocial factors;
- Applying basic control methods to reduce the total exposure duration, frequency and dose of the risk factor should be part of the training for the hypermobile individual;
- Postural education for dynamic tasks (e.g. lifting, pushing, pulling) and static tasks (e.g. sitting, standing, holding tools, interacting with work equipment);
- The importance of early reporting of symptoms and intervention;
- Encouragement to attend specialist physical training (under the guidance of their clinician) to improve the recruitment of core stability muscles, joint proprioception and kinaesthesia (movement awareness) may be of benefit;
- Ensuring task cycle breaks to reduce postural muscle fatigue.

Should the individual find that their threshold for mental demand or stress is potentially affected by chronic pain or disability, the psychological demands of the task must be considered. Such psychosocial factors as total workload, time constraints, lack of autonomy, lack of performance feedback and control over their job must be considered and evaluated by the ergonomist.

Ergonomic assessment and management

The ergonomist is encouraged to work closely with the individual and the employer to provide a systematic subjective and objective assessment of the individual's status and job requirements. Analysis of the findings and synthesis of potential problems should follow, so that realistic recommendations to reduce the risk factors may be put forward. Appendix I provides an example of an ergonomic assessment form used for those who require individual consultation and specific recommendations. The reader will note that photographs are sometimes used to present the scenario much more clearly. Those approving and implementing the recommendations usually find the pictures particularly helpful.

Follow-up after implementation of the control measures is essential. It is also recommended that all ergonomic interventions be trialled prior to being accepted as the final solution.

Should permission be provided by the individual, it may be highly beneficial for the ergonomist to liaise with their clinician (medical doctor or physiotherapist) to obtain a greater understanding of the individual's condition and provide feedback about the workplace findings. Hales and Bertsche (1999) state that open lines of communication between employer, employee and the healthcare provider are essential. Attending combined clinics may be particularly valuable for all parties involved (e.g. combined upper limb clinic at the University College London Hospitals, Rheumatology Department, attended by patient, rheumatologist, therapist and ergonomist).

Secondary prevention

Job restrictions and task modifications

Employees returning to the same job without modification of the work environment are at risk of recurrence (Hales and Bertsche 1999). The principles guiding the return to work include the type of WRMSD, the severity of the condition and the risk factor present on the job. Following injury or presentation of problems, it is highly beneficial for the ergonomist to work closely with the clinician, should permission be provided by the patient. Understanding the pathology, tissue mechanics and working diagnosis allows the ergonomist to analyse the individual's task more specifically and reduce those risk factors that may be related to the condition presented. For example, a hypermobile individual may present with right shoulder instability and scapulothoracic pain, especially aggravated by computer use. Closer analysis of their task may reveal that intensive mouse use in a non-neutral shoulder position is evident. Initially, the individual may be encouraged to avoid mouse – and possibly keyboard – use by carrying out alternative dynamic tasks (e.g. writing and filing). As the individual recovers from the acute condition, recommendations such as the avoidance of intensive right upper limb mouse use (e.g. substitution by keystrokes, or left-hand mouse use), postural training at the workplace, trying an alternative keyboard design (which does not have a number pad attached to the right, which would normally restrict mouse placement) and trying an alternative mouse design (e.g. a touchpad mouse, which does not require static shoulder girdle contraction) may be suggested. The workplace findings and recommendations may also provide the clinician with further understanding about the pathogenesis of the individual's condition, and ideas for therapy (e.g. utilizing EMG biofeedback to train the individual to recruit lower trapezius for improved shoulder stability and muscle balance, or using proprioceptive neuromuscular therapy to regain normal proprioception and kinaesthesia of the upper quadrant).

Education and training to prevent persistence or recurrence of injury

It is imperative that the hypermobile individual understands what the potential work-related factors that may have aggravated their musculoskeletal condition are, so that exposure to them may be reduced or avoided altogether. The ergonomist who has a full understanding of the individual's condition may be the practitioner best placed to provide this advice, as they may be most familiar with the particular risk factors.

Ergonomic assessment and management

Ergonomic assessments following injury or the presentation of symptoms (reactive ergonomics) may reduce the scope of the assessment but increase its detail, as high-priority factors to be corrected are usually revealed more readily. General prophylactic ergonomic risk assessments tend to require the ergonomist to think in a broad and proactive manner, considering all factors that may pose as risks. Appendix 9.1 presents an ergonomic assessment form which may be used at all levels of prevention.

Tertiary prevention

Rehabilitation and gradual return to work/conditioning

Scientists confirm that rehabilitation and ergonomics applied together considerably intensify and advance both the progress of the rehabilitation process and the return to normal life (Nowak 1999).

Returning injured or disabled workers to the workforce through accommodations and redesign of the work environment and tasks is possible only with sufficient information about the physical and cognitive requirements of the task (Mayer et al. 2000). A detailed ergonomic assessment would usually reveal the requirements and physical capacity of the individual. The latter may not be easily obvious in the work setting, as psychosocial factors and fear of reinjury may prevent the individual from working at their actual physical capability. Functional capacity examinations (e.g. Key and Blankenship methods) may provide the ergonomist with subjective and objective measures of the individual's capacity. However, the application of the objective measures may be limited, because for many the information has been collected within a controlled, rather than a natural work environment.

Providing the injured worker with a job with modified tasks during rehabilitation or following physical impairment will allow them to maintain their function and often promote positive perceptions about their capabilities. It is important that the modified task be one that is required for normal or improved function for the organization (rather than created for the individual, without particular benefit to the organization), so that the individual may feel valued and functional on their return to work. Clinicians must advise which tasks should be avoided, at various progressive stages of tissue healing or rehabilitation. Gradual increase of endurance is important not only for improving total muscular strength and power, but also for adaptation to new and controlled patterns of movement (demands of proprioception and kinaesthesia). Regular attendance at a workplace will often require social interaction, and may reduce the risk of the individual falling into the trap of perceiving themselves as having a permanent disability.

Ergonomic assessment and management

Striking a balance between physical limitations and job requirements requires a detailed understanding and recognition of all elements on either side of the balance. The ergonomic assessment must usually be carried out with high sensitivity, so that progression to return to work can be accepted rather than rejected by the individual. Should the individual be unwilling to increase their function, because of either fear of physical reinjury or increased social interaction within the workplace, then the ergonomist must recognize this early on. With consent of the individual, a multidisciplinary approach (possibly with input from the medical doctor, physiotherapist, occupational therapist, psychologist, vocational rehabilitation specialist) with commitment by the individual's employer may be required for these situations. Maintaining objectivity during the assessment and presenting realistic goals is especially important.

CONCLUSION

The prevalence of musculoskeletal disorders in the workplace is high. The causes are thought to be multifactorial and include repetitive movement, the force involved, awkward and static postures, vibration, temperature and psychosocial issues. It is important to have an appreciation of the biological responses and possible pathologies that can result from these factors in order to manage symptoms successfully. This is particularly relevant in the hypermobile individual, who is possibly more at risk because of their more vulnerable tissues. The application of ergonomic principles is essential to prevent the development of musculoskeletal problems and successfully manage problems when they arise.

REFERENCES

Adams, M.A. and Hutton, W.C. (1982) Prolapsed intervertebral disc: a hyperflexion injury. *Spine*, **7**, 184–91.

Armstrong, T., Castelli, W., Evans, G. and Dias-Perez, R. (1984) Some histological changes in carpal tunnel contents and their biomechanical implications. *Journal of Occupational Medicine*, **26**, 197–201.

Armstrong, T.J., Buckle, P., Fine, L.J. et al. (1993) A conceptual model for work-related neck and upper-limb musculoskeletal disorders. *Scandinavian Journal of Work Environment and Health*, **19**, 73–84.

Ashton-Miller, J.A. (1999) Response of muscle and tendon injury and overuse. In: *Work Related Musculoskeletal Disorders: Report, Workshop Summary and Workshop Papers.* National Research Council, pp. 73–97. National Academy Press.

Backman, C., Boquist, L., Friden, J. et al. (1990) Chronic Achilles paratendonitis with tendinosis: an experimental model in the rabbit. *Journal of Orthopaedic Research*, **8**, 541–54.

Beighton, P.H., Grahame, R. and Bird, H.A. (1998) *Hypermobility of Joints*, 3rd edn. Springer-Verlag.

Bovenzi, M. (2000) Health disorders caused by occupational exposure to vibration. In: *Occupational Ergonomics: Work Related Musculoskeletal Disorders of The Upper Limb and Back* (F. Violante, T. Armstrong and A. Kilbom, eds), pp. 89–104. Taylor and Francis.

Chaffin, D.B. and Andersen, G.B.J. (1991) *Occupational Biomechanics*. New York: John Wiley and Sons.

Edwards, R.H.T. (1988) Hypothesis of peripheral and central mechanisms underlying occupational muscle pain and injury. *European Journal of Applied Physiology and Occupational Physiology*, **57**, 275–81.

European Agency for Safety and Health at Work (EASHW) (1999) *Work-Related Neck and Upper Limb Musculoskeletal Disorders*. Office for Official Publications of the European Communities.

Garcia-Cruz, D., Cano-Colin, S., Sanchez-Corona, J. et al. (1998) Clinical, morphological and biochemical features in the familial articular hypermobility syndrome (FAHS): a family study. *Clinical Genetics*, **53**, 108–13.

Goldstein S., Armstrong T., Chaffin, D. and Matthews, L. (1987) Analysis of cumulative strain in tendons and tendon sheaths. *Journal of Biomechanics*, **20**, 1–6.

Grahame, R. (2000) Pain, distress and joint hyperlaxity. *Joint Bone Spine*, **67**, 157–63.

Grandjean, E. (1982) *Fitting the Task to the Man: an Ergonomic Approach*. Taylor and Francis.

Haberhauer, G., Feyertag, J., Hanusch-Enserer, U. and Dunky, A. (2000) Joint hypermobility syndrome and bilateral total occlusion of the ulnar arteries presenting as Raynaud's phenomenon. *Clinical and Experimental Rheumatology*, **18**, 270–1.

Hagberg, M. and Hagberg, C. (1989) Risks and prevention of musculoskeletal disorders among dentists. In: *Occupational Hazards in the Health Professions* (D.K. Brune and C. Edling, eds), pp. 323–32. CRC Press.

Hales, T. and Bertsche, P. (1999) Medical management of work-related musculoskeletal disorders. In: *The Occupational Ergonomics Handbook* (W. Karwowski and W.S. Marras, eds), pp. 1333–52. CRC Press.

Hall, M.G., Ferrell, W.R., Sturock, R.D., Hamblen, D.L. and Baxendale, R.H. (1995) The effect of the hypermobility syndrome on knee joint proprioception. *British Journal of Rheumatology*, **34**, 121–5.

Hägg, G. (1998, cited in EASHW, 1999) Muscle fibre abnormalities in the upper trapezius muscle related to occupational static load. International Conference in Occupational Disorders of the Upper Extremities, 10–11 December, Burlingame,
California, University of Michigan and the University of California.

Howes, J. and Isdale, I.C. (1971) The loose back: an unrecognised syndrome. *Rheumatology and Physical Medicine*, **11**, 72–7.

Ireland, D. (1995) *Cumulative Trauma Disorders of the Upper Extremity: II, American Association for Hand Surgeons Conference Proceedings*, August 1995, American Association for Hand Surgeons.

Jonsson, B. (1982) Measurement and evaluation of local muscular strain on the shoulder during constrained work. *Journal of Human Ergology*, **11**, 73–88.

Khalil, T.M., Abdel-Moty, E., Steele-Rosomoff, R. and Rosomoff, H. (1999) Ergonomic programs in post injury management. In: *The Occupational Ergonomics Handbook* (W. Karwowski and W.S. Marras, eds), pp. 1333–52. Boca Raton: CRC Press.

Kumar, S. (2001) Theories of musculoskeletal injury causation. *Ergonomics*, **44**(1): 17–47.

Larsson, L., Mudholkar, G.S., Baum, J. and Srivastava, D.K. (1995) Benefits and liabilities of hypermobility in the back pain disorders of industrial workers. *Journal of Internal Medicine*, **238**, 461–7.

Larsson, L., Baum, J., Mudholkar, G.S. and Kollia, G.D. (1993) Benefits and disadvantages of joint hypermobility among musicians. *New England Journal of Medicine*, **329**, 1079–82.

MacDonald, L.A., Karasek, R.A., Punnett, L. and Scharf T. (2001) Covariation between workplace physical and psychosocial stressors: evidence and implications for occupational health research and prevention. *Ergonomics*, **10**, 696–718.

Magnusson, S.P., Julsgaard, C., Aagaard, P. et al. (2001) Viscoelastic properties and flexibility of the human muscle–tendon unit in benign joint hypermobility syndrome. *Journal of Rheumatology*, **28**, 2720–5.

March, L. and Silman, A. (1993) Joint hyperlaxity: is there a case for screening? *British Journal of Rheumatology*, **32**, 91–2.

Mayer, T.G., Gatchel, R.J. and Polatin, P.B. (2000) *Occupational Musculoskeletal Disorders: Function, Outcomes and Evidence*. Lippincott, Williams & Wilkins.

Melin, B. and Lundberg, U. (1997) A biopsychosocial approach to work-stress and musculoskeletal disorders. *Journal of Psychophysiology*, **11**, 238–47.

Miller, E.J. and Gay, S. (1987) The collagens: an overview and update. *Methods in Enzymology*, **144**, 3–43.

Mishra, M.B., Ryan, P. and Atkinson, P. (1996) Extra-articular features of benign joint hypermobility syndrome. *British Journal of Rheumatology*, **35**, 861–6.

National Research Council (1999) *Work Related Musculoskeletal Disorders: Report, Workshop Summary and Workshop Papers.* National Academy Press.

National Research Council and Institute of Medicine (2001) *Musculoskeletal Disorders and the Workplace.* National Academy Press.

Nijs, J., van Essche, E., De Munck, M. and Dequeker, J. (2000) Ultrasonographic, axial and peripheral measurements in female patients with benign hypermobility syndrome. *Calcified Tissue International*, **67**, 37–40.

NIOSH (1997) *Musculoskeletal Disorders and Workplace Factors.* National Institute for Occupational Safety and Health.

Nowak, E. (1999) Ergonomics and rehabilitation. In: *The Occupational Ergonomics Handbook.* (W. Karwowski and W.S. Marras, eds), pp. 1333–52. Boca Raton: CRC Press.

Oliver, J. and Middleditch, A. (2000) *Functional Anatomy of the Spine.* Butterworth–Heinemann.

Pope, M., De Vocht, J.W., McIntyre, D.R. and Marker, T.K. (2000) The thoracolumbar spine. In: *Occupational Musculoskeletal Disorders* (T.G. Mayer, R.J. Gatchel and P.B. Polatin, eds), pp. 65–81. Lippincott, Williams & Wilkins.

Radwin, R.G. and Lavender, S.A. (1999) Work factors, personal factors and internal loads: biomechanics of work stressors. In: *Work Related Musculoskeletal Disorders: Report, Workshop Summary and Workshop Papers.* National Research Council, pp. 98–115. National Academy Press.

Sahrmann, S. (2002) *Diagnosis and Treatment of Movement Impairment Syndromes.* Mosby.

Sharma, L. (1999) Proprioceptive impairment in knee osteoarthritis. *Rheumatic Disease Clinics of North America*, **25**, 299–314.

Sharma, L. and Pai Y.C. (1997) Impaired proprioception and osteoarthritis. *Current Opinion in Rheumatology*, **9**, 253–8.

Silverman, S., Constine, L., Harvey, W. and Grahame, R. (1975) Survey of joint mobility and in vivo skin elasticity in London schoolchildren. *Annals of the Rheumatic Diseases*, **34**, 177–80.

Straker, L.M., Pollock, C.M. and Mangharam, J. (1997) The effect of shoulder posture on performance, discomfort and muscle fatigue whilst working on a visual display unit. *International Journal of Industrial Ergonomics*, **20**, 1–10.

Veiersted, K.B., Westgaard, R.H. and Andersen, P. (1993) Electromyographic evaluation of muscular pattern as a predictor of trapezius myalgia. *Scandinavian Journal of Work Environment and Health*, **19**, 284–90.

Violante, R., Armstrong, T. and Kilbom, A. (2000) *Occupational Ergonomics: Work-Related Musculoskeletal Disorders of the Upper Limb and Back.* London: Taylor and Francis.

Waersted, M. and Westgaard, R.H. (1996) Attention related muscle activity in different body regions during VDU work with minimal physical activity. *Ergonomics*, **39**, 661–76.

Appendix 9.1

INDIVIDUAL ERGONOMIC ASSESSMENT

Personal information

Date:	Ergonomic assessor:
Client name	
Gender	
Date of birth	
Employer/company	
Job title	
Business unit/department	
Manager/contact person	
Work location	
Relevant past medical history (stated by client)	

Subjective assessment (reported by client)

Work status: Full-time/Part-time/Permanent/Temporary/Trainee

Restrictions: Full duty/restricted duty/awaiting to return to work

Length of working day:

Frequency and periods of breaks (scheduled and natural):

Scheduled breaks:

Natural breaks:

Job description and designated tasks

Task	Description (% keyboard, mouse, screen, telephone, writing where applicable)

Current relevant presenting complaints:

Mobility of client: Wheelchair /walking with aids/walking independently

If client ambulates, is there a limitation?

Objective assessment (assessor's findings)

Primary workstation layout
(PHOTOS OR SKETCH)

Primary tasks observed

	Repetitive movement (high/ medium/ low)	Static postures (high/ medium/ low)	Awkward postures (high/ medium/ low)	Extreme forces exerted (high/ medium/ low)	Contact stress (high/ medium/ low)	Vibration (high/ medium/ low)

Equipment measures (mm) (e.g. in office setting)

Equipment type and model if obvious: Desk: Chair: Mouse: Keyboard: VDU: Other equipment:
Seat-pan height:
Seat pan width × depth:
Lumbar support height:
Back rest width × length:
Desk height:
Desk thickness:
Keyboard height:
Screen size (diagonal length):
Top of screen height:
Screen depth from eye:

Anthropometric measures (mm)

Anthropometric measures
Height:
Weight:
R/L-handed:
Knee height (heel to popliteus/top):
Mid-thigh height:
Hip height (joint):
Lumbar lordosis height (seat pan to lordosis):
Hips width:
Thigh length in sitting (buttock to popliteus):
Elbow height (seat pan to elbow):
Torso length (buttock to shoulder height in sitting):
Sitting eye height (seat pan to eyes):
Funct. reach length:

Health and safety

Yes   No

Has a risk assessment been carried out at your workstation?
Have you received training related to health and safety?

Environmental conditions

	Acceptable to client	Not acceptable to client (briefly state issue) – recommended to be assessed by employer
Lighting conditions		
Observed general hygiene level		
Observed slips, trips, falls, hazards		
Current noise level		
Current air quality		
Current temperature		

Problems identified
1.
2.
etc.

Recommendations

Equipment

Equipment recommendation
Rationale
Details of installation and training requirements
Suppliers

Access

Access recommendation
Rationale

Workstation layout

Workstation layout recommendation
Rationale

Recommended workstation layout
(SKETCH)

Training – postural re-education and work practice

Training recommendation
Rationale

Task redesign

Task redesign recommendation
Rationale
Agreed by client

Other comments

Assessor's signature: _____

Printed name (qualifications): _____

Date: _____

(Developed by Jean Mangharam for ErgoSense Ltd, 2000)

10

Joint hypermobility and chronic pain: possible linking mechanisms and management highlighted by a cognitive–behavioural approach

Vicki Harding

Aims

1. To explore the possible links between chronic pain and joint hypermobility
2. To discuss why patients with symptomatic joint hypermobility may become chronic pain patients
3. To discuss the management of hypermobile patients with chronic pain using a cognitive–behavioural approach
4. To explore the impact that unhelpful beliefs on the part of the patient and the medical profession have on the management of chronic pain

---

INTRODUCTION

Are those with joint hypermobility syndrome (JHS) predisposed to having pain and, if so, what might the mechanisms be? This is a question that must have frequently been considered by rheumatologists, physiotherapists and others who regularly come across people with JHS in their clinics. It is easy to surmise that the two conditions are linked. Previous chapters have described some new research linking joint hypermobility with various interesting clinical and neurobiological phenomena. The literature, however, has not yet provided strong evidence for cause and effect. Neither has it indicated with any certainty what the linking mechanisms between pain and hypermobility might be, why joint hypermobility might predispose one to having a chronic pain condition, and why some people with hypermobile joints go on to have JHS and others do not.

Chronic pain management using an interdisciplinary cognitive–behavioural approach has been functioning in the UK since the mid to late 1980s. This form of pain management takes a biopsychosocial approach, rather than a purely tissue-based diagnostic approach. As such, although it has been found to be useful for most pain conditions, it will be very helpful for pain patients with gaps in understanding of the pain mechanisms operating in their particular condition. Because the cognitive–behavioural approach uses a normal learning rather than a pathological model, it looks at the way people's patterns of thinking and function affect their ability to cope with pain. It then goes on to use this knowledge to inform their approach to learning more effective coping and ways of improving and broadening their physical function. It helps them to understand and come to terms with the chronicity of their pain, teaches them ways of improving their mood in spite of their pain, and how to cope with pain flare-ups and more difficult times.

The author already had an interest in joint hypermobility when she helped set up the largest pain management programme in the UK in 1988, the INPUT unit at St Thomas' Hospital, London. Her experience in chronic pain management has enabled her to see certain patterns emerge for those with either just hypermobile joints or full-blown JHS, explaining why pain management is so helpful for them in managing their pain. This chapter will describe some of the features of her experience with chronic pain and JHS/joint hypermobility that may provide some help in managing this complex and burdensome duo.

LINKS BETWEEN CHRONIC PAIN AND JOINT HYPERMOBILITY

Joint hypermobility is a trait that for many – and possibly most – individuals gives rise to no symptoms or difficulties. For some individuals joint hypermobility merely means they are at one extreme of a normal range. For others, however, it appears that joint hypermobility can give rise to a level of problems that is over and above what might be considered to be a normal incidence of common musculoskeletal problems in the wider population. The Guy's Hospital studies (Grahame et al. 1981, Mishra et al. 1996) have proffered evidence that indicates that JHS is an, albeit mild, heritable connective disorder of collagen (probably identical with the EDS hypermobility type, formerly EDS III), though it can easily be distinguished on clinical grounds from such disorders as EDS classic type, formerly EDS I and II, and Marfan syndrome (Grahame 1999). Even for those whose hypermobility gives them an advantage, such as musicians, dancers and swimmers, it is suggested that this advantage should still be seen in the context of understanding the needs and limits of the individual's particular collagenous tissues.

One of the clues that some with joint hypermobility do have extra problems is found in the chronic pain population. Anecdotal reports from clinicians with an interest in joint hypermobility in rheumatology clinics, physiotherapy departments and chronic pain management units, indicate that such patients appear to form a much larger proportion of the chronic pain population than would be expected. The literature is rather confusing, as some find there is no significant difference in hypermobility incidence between subjects with or without pain. Fairbank and colleagues (1984) found no difference in the incidence of hypermobility between 310 children with no pain and 136 with anterior knee pain, whereas others do. Gedalia and colleagues (1985) found that 12% of 260 normal schoolchildren but 66% of 66 children with juvenile episodic arthritis had joint hypermobility. In 1993, Gedalia and colleagues went on to find that in a group of 338 school children 13% had joint hypermobility and 6% had fibromyalgia, but 81% of those with fibromyalgia had joint hypermobility. In a Finnish study of 1637 preadolescents there was no difference in the incidence of musculoskeletal pain in those with a Beighton score of ≥6/9 and those who were designated 'non-hypermobile' (presumably ≤5/9) (Mikkelsson et al. 1963). By contrast, in a group of young adult army recruits there was a highly significant association between hypermobility and the occurrence of traumatic soft tissue lesions (Acasuso et al. 1994).

Most patients attending the INPUT pain management programme are quite severely disabled by their pain, and one important feature that is noticeable is their *lack* of mobility, complaints of stiffness, and reduced functional range of motion – for many quite extreme – following years of inactivity. Standard signs of joint hypermobility, however, are present in many of our chronic pain patients. The texture and increased stretchiness of their skin seems to indicate a connective tissue disorder, and it is particularly noticeable that these patients' postures commonly have that quality of grace and drape that is characteristic of hypermobile subjects. Their children too, when they come for 'friends and family' sessions, also demonstrate this, as can be seen in Figure 10.1.

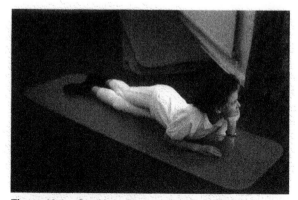

Figure 10.1   Qualities of postural grace and drape observed in a family member.

THE PROPORTION OF PEOPLE WITH JOINT HYPERMOBILITY IN A CHRONIC PAIN POPULATION

Assessing the incidence of joint hypermobility in a population is not easy, not least because the standard methods of scoring for joint hypermobility – the Beighton (Beighton et al. 1973) and Contompasis (McNerny and Johnston 1979) scoring systems – have not undergone systematic reliability testing, though Bulbena et al. (1992) have shown good correlation between the various available scoring systems. In addition, many people stiffen up as they reduce their activity levels or avoid stretching, as can occur when people take more sedentary jobs or experience pain. However, in an initial pilot study of 36 Caucasian INPUT patients (Harding and Grahame 1990), seven people (19.4%) scored ≥4 on the Beighton scoring system. In addition, 18 (50%) reported being able in the past to place their hands flat on the floor when bending over with their knees straight. Fifteen (41.6%) of these also reported a family history of hypermobility, or that they were able to perform contortions when younger. One was even part of a family of 13 professional contortionists – 11 brothers and sisters and both parents!

When collagen analysis and genetic testing become more freely available, and more is known about the markers for hypermobility, then more precise population studies will be possible. Until then, it is only possible to suggest trends in the context of only poor to moderate measurement reliability. Nevertheless, even if an estimate of 4–7% in the white Caucasian population is considered conservative, and given the relative unreliability of the measures available at present, it is difficult to dispute that the incidence of joint hypermobility is raised in the chronic pain population seeking help. At INPUT it would appear that up to approximately 40% of our chronic pain patients could be deemed as having past or present joint hypermobility, though it should be emphasized that this is made up of patients with JHS and others with chronic pain but without JHS.

The pilot study, though small, certainly suggested that the incidence was substantially higher than that expected in the general population.

POSSIBLE REASONS FOR THE HIGH INCIDENCE OF JOINT HYPERMOBILITY IN A CHRONIC PAIN POPULATION, THAT GIVE INSIGHT INTO MANAGEMENT

Joint hypermobility is a relatively common trait and so may have conferred some evolutionary advantage. Now that humans no longer live as hunter–gatherers, this evolutionary advantage may no longer be operating within some of the conditions that either optimize it or prevent any disadvantage that it brings – such as pain – emerging. There is currently little in the literature to indicate why hypermobility and chronic pain would be linked. Bulbena and colleagues from Spain, however, have demonstrated a chromosomal duplication linking joint laxity with anxiety and panic (Bulbena et al. 1993, Gratacos et al. 2001). Because chronic pain patients are naturally more disabled and distressed than pain-free populations this is an interesting link. Because INPUT was set up as a research project, patients were measured over a range of demographic, medical, physical function and psychological parameters. However, in the 36 INPUT patients studied above, the hypermobile patients could not be distinguished from the non-hypermobile patients in terms of their level of anxiety as measured with the State Trait Anxiety Inventory (STAI) (Spielberger 1983). Subjects who were hypermobile or had a history of hypermobility scored a mean of 48.3 (SD 11.9) on the STAI, whereas those without current or historical joint hypermobility scored a mean of 48.7 (SD 14.2). There was thus no significant difference in anxiety between them, both being a little raised, as might be expected considering they had had their pain for a mean of 9.8 years and were still seeking treatment. These data are as yet unpublished, and further work is needed to establish whether the anxiety is indeed a primary feature of joint hypermobility or merely a secondary effect of having a long-term, painful but unexplained condition. It would also seem valuable to repeat this study but compare those with JHS with other chronic pain subjects, rather than merely comparing chronic pain patients with and without joint hypermobility.

Certainly there is as yet no established and demonstrated single *causative* link between joint hypermobility and chronic pain reported in the literature. Considering the many factors involved in the predisposition, causation and maintenance of chronic pain, and the heterogeneity of joint hypermobility, it is likely that the factors linking joint hypermobility and chronic pain are also likely to be multiple, most probably with complex interactions, requiring a large number of patients to establish possible links and interactions. There are, however, some clues emerging from clinical experience in pain management as to what contributing factors may play a part, which also point to their appropriate management.

Chronic pain is a complex syndrome, with probably as many combinations of causative factors, patient responses and maintaining factors as there are patients. Nevertheless, there are many common difficulties that chronic pain sufferers have (Harding 1998, Main and Spanswick 2000, Williams and Erskine 1995) to a greater or lesser degree. These include:

- Patterns of overactivity/underactivity cycling;
- Use of a tissue damage model;
- Lack of helpful information;
- Unhelpful beliefs or cognitive styles.

It can be speculated that the high incidence of joint hypermobility in this population would tend to indicate that difficulties frequently encountered by chronic pain patients are likely to include factors that are particularly pertinent for hypermobile subjects and a clue to the more important maintaining or aetiological factors for this group.

Equally, if pain management is effective, it can be argued that factors contributing to its effectiveness are likely to include those that are also pertinent to hypermobility. The published data on the outcome of pain management are impressive. Flor et al.'s (1992) meta-analysis of 65 studies showed that even at long-term follow-up, patients are functioning better than 75% of a sample who were either untreated or treated by conventional methods. Morley et al. (1999), in their systematic review, determined that patients treated by cognitive–behavioural methods fared significantly better than waiting list controls and those on other treatments.

Despite the evidence of efficacy for cognitive–behavioural pain management, there is at present no definitive evidence as to which factors are important for hypermobile subjects. Patients with joint hypermobility who are attending pain management clinics, however, and therapists working in pain management, are suggesting some important areas that are worth considering. These are discussed in the following sections.

DIAGNOSIS

For hypermobile patients, understanding their diagnosis can be a problem. Some have been given a diagnosis and explanation and accept that this of itself can cause chronic pain. However, there are still some hypermobile patients who do not yet have a definitive diagnosis and share some of the diagnosis-related problems common to other chronic pain patients:

- There are no laboratory tests that can validate the report of pain in people with joint hypermobility.
- Patients and their doctors often still have a tissue-damage approach to the diagnosis, rather than a biopsychosocial one. Many doctors and therapists still find it difficult to explain the neurophysiology of chronic pain to their patients, or do not understand it themselves.

Without this it is almost impossible for them to understand what the patient is experiencing, or at least justify to the patient's satisfaction the level of pain.
- Treatments for the pain have on the whole been ineffective, or even made the pain worse, which again can create doubt in patients' or their doctors' minds about aetiology: 'Well, *why* isn't it getting better, *why* can't they do something?'
- Not having a name for their condition that makes the pain readily explicable makes it difficult to ask for help from others, and can create major problems at work or with Social Security benefit agencies.
- Others can hint or suggest that since there is no clear cause, the pain might be 'in their mind', and even patients themselves can begin to doubt their sanity.
- Not having a discrete injury to mark the onset of pain can make it particularly harrowing to undergo Department of Work and Pensions (DWP) (formerly DSS) interviews or examinations, where the message may be that they have nothing wrong with them.
- Even if there was an injury at the outset, it is still mystifying to patients and their families as to why their symptoms have not got better. Again, it can sometimes be implied that the patient somehow doesn't 'want' to get better.
- Not knowing, understanding or being believed can become a very great burden, even when patients themselves have come to terms with the fact that the pain is long term.

Many chronic pain patients report that they do not feel believed. One particular factor that patients with hypermobility have to contend with is that they are not obviously limited in their movement. This can lead to some feeling dismissed, as if their pain is not serious: 'When that one said "I can't touch my toes, there's nothing wrong with you" I felt so angry, but I also felt really put down. Do they expect me to fake things?'

In addition to diagnostic issues, various beliefs about pain can also lead to increased disability or have an effect on mood:

- Pain means damage – 'If doing something hurts I should avoid it'.
- 'I'll get worse as I get older – it's hopeless, maybe I should just accept I'll end up in a wheelchair, but I don't want to'.
- 'Even my "good" side is hurting now – it's taking too much strain making up for the "bad" side'.
- 'I've got wear and tear – better not use my joints/spine or they'll wear out even quicker'.
- 'If the pain gets any worse I'll go mad – I'm desperate, surely no-one could be expected to cope with this?'
- 'I need to rest more – if you feel tired it means you've been doing too much. You should rest until you feel better'.
- 'If I can just wait long enough, someone will be able to do something – surely they'll discover the cure for pain soon: modern medicine is working miracles these days'.
- 'My pain is a sign of whether I am better. I won't be better until my pain has gone'.

Although these unhelpful beliefs occur frequently for many chronic pain patients, those with joint hypermobility may also have other concerns and beliefs, such as:

- 'I'm too mobile, I might put my joints out if I do too much – I should avoid any stretching.'
- 'If you are hypermobile your joints fall apart when you get older/I shall get crippled with arthritis.'
- 'Doing ballet/gymnastics damaged my joints because I'm too supple.'

If these beliefs are allowed to continue, then teaching patients how to improve their coping skills is likely to be ineffective as they may regard them as trivial or irrelevant compared with their expectations of or hopes for medical treatment. Their fears may also undermine any sense of achievement. Addressing erroneous beliefs with interactive information sessions, providing patients with evidence of the ability of their joints to improve through paced activity, and teaching cognitive strategies to challenge unhelpful cognitive patterns such as all-or-nothing thinking, are effective in helping patients to make changes.

OVERACTIVITY–UNDERACTIVITY CYCLING AND PACING

Overactivity–underactivity cycling is common to virtually all those attending chronic pain management clinics (Harding 1998) and is a major cause of pain flare-ups. Furthermore, many hypermobile subjects also seem to suffer more 'training' pain than those without joint hypermobility, even if they do not have chronic pain: 'If we climb a hill, or play tennis together, I pay more for it than my partner does'. It is easy to speculate that those with joint hypermobility are 'good' at stretch and thus not very good at strengthening or endurance, just as those we know who seem to have been born with 'stiff genes' hate stretching but are very good at weight-lifting and endurance pursuits.

It is important not to emphasize to patients a sense of weakness, inadequacy or friability of their tissue, but to refer to them as on a continuum whereby for them their collagenous tissues are easier to stretch, but take more persistent work to strengthen and toughen. Even for those with Ehlers–Danlos syndrome, whose tissue is more friable, it is still nevertheless possible to place the emphasis on maximizing tissue health and strength. Otherwise, it can be possible for them only to see a bleak future where they are at the mercy of their tissues. This is likely to lead to loss of fitness and deconditioning as they avoid putting 'strain' on their tissues, resulting in further deterioration.

What is clear is that pacing is vital to those with hypermobility, who find it hard to strengthen or take part in activities requiring endurance, but in whom building up their strength and endurance is important. This means using a systematic graded approach from a baseline, and spacing out and varying activities. As reported elsewhere (Harding 1998), pacing is established by first setting the baseline for the activity. A baseline is an amount that can be 'easily manageable', that is, pain may or may not be present or induced, but is easily manageable if it is. This should also be the level at which confidence (or lack of it) is easily manageable and effort reduced to a minimum. This is a difficult concept for many who are used to doing most activities at their maximum effort, so even reducing a little should be seen as improvement and the patient encouraged to try even less the next time. As pain at the time of activity is not a useful guide to setting a baseline, with pain flare-ups usually coming some time afterwards, it is advisable to try several baselines over several days. This allows patients to be ultracautious the first day, as they can always go up a little the next day, but if they still get subsequent unmanageable pain at least this is minimized and they can try less or use less effort the next time. The concept of a 'homeopathic exercise' if the person's fear or pain is such that they are unable to start with even easy versions of exercises or activities can be helpful.

Measurement is taken by counting exercises or activities, or by timing them with an electronic timer. A good rule is for patients to make two or three baseline measurements of each exercise or activity, ideally at different times of the day; they are then taught to average these measurements and start at 80% of the average. This reduces the risk that they may be starting too high, helps build confidence, and means that conceptually patients will feel more able to keep to their quota on a 'bad' day. If a patient has had a problem for many years there is no need to rush towards achieving high levels of activity or fitness. It is more important that patients learn *how* to do it, as they can then continue the process themselves over a more realistic time span. Pacing up then follows, with patients generally setting their own pacing rate once a week, at a level that they can easily maintain for that week. A general rule of thumb is to encourage patients to pace up at *less* than 10% a day. On the whole, patients will pace up more slowly than that. For some activities it may be necessary to build by one exercise a week until confidence increases sufficiently for them to build up a little faster. Different activities will require different pacing rates, activities producing the more persistent or severe pain taking considerably longer. The general trend in improvement for most tasks is usually logarithmic – faster improvement is seen early on, which then gradually slows until after some months it almost plateaus off. Pacing will also fluctuate from week to week according to pain flare-ups and changes in mood and confidence levels, but because it is set weekly the patient remains in control rather than allowing their symptoms to do so. Clinical experience suggests that those with joint hypermobility need to pace up more slowly on strengthening and endurance activities, but there is as yet no evidence base for this. It is vital that patients use a timer for pacing their activities. This is the only way to ensure they are systematic in their increase, using quota completion rather than pain as a guide as to when to stop, with the beeper preventing them forgetting or being 'carried away'! Vibration timers, originally produced for the deaf, are available for those whose work or circumstances would find the beeper too intrusive (from SarabeC; 01642 247789, email: http//www.sarabec.co.uk).

Movement variety is the other arm of pacing. This involves many parameters, including changing between more active and more sedentary tasks, and between more flexed or more extended joint postures, as well as between those activities that use more relaxed or more intense muscle work, closer precision work or grosser movements. Even those for whom hypermobility is an advantage for their profession or sport still need to ensure that they balance flexibility with strength and endurance, and pace this up systematically and gradually, allowing consideration for their collagen, and aiming to minimize training pain. This approach is generally likely to minimize the risk of injury, ensuring that fitness does not peak too early and maintains well. In the early days, while fitness and tolerances for activities such as sitting and walking are low, very frequent changes need to be made. As these build up, changes will reduce in frequency and feel less intrusive.

Patients attending INPUT with the classic form of Ehlers–Danlos syndrome have demonstrated the importance of pacing static positions. Any tissue with elastic properties likes stretch, but prolonged stretch causes fibre failure, such as occurs with the skin stretch marks of pregnancy. The ligaments of the interphalangeal joints, for example, can take the weight of the body and more when the person hangs from a tree branch by their fingers. Even with very strong muscles, however, this cannot be maintained as a static stretch for long, as pain receptors in the ligament attachments prevent prolonged stretch from causing damage. It is easy to speculate that those with Ehlers–Danlos syndrome might be more susceptible to prolonged stretching of their collagen because of its greater extensibility: for example their greater susceptibility to pes planus following prolonged standing. Indeed, these patients do seem generally to be more uncomfortable in static postures, with shorter tolerances, and are often already 'spacing' – taking regular breaks or changes of position, often cleverly disguised. Pacing these postures more carefully to build tolerance but preventing overuse by using a timer, does eventually allow their tolerance for these postures to build and pain flare-ups to reduce. For Ehlers–Danlos syndrome though, we advise that they keep their time goals for these postures still relatively short and try to maintain good body mechanics with joint support in neutral positions, interspersed with more aerobic, circulation-boosting activity to ensure healthy tissues. An example of this was a teacher with Ehlers–Danlos syndrome who adapted her teaching methods to prevent standing for long periods at the blackboard, broke up her long journey across London to work, negotiated three short lying-down rest breaks, and went for a brisk walk during her lunch break to help her cope. Although not in the same league as those with classic Ehlers–Danlos syndrome, some patients with joint hypermobility, particularly those with JHS, have echoes of their discomfort and low tolerances for static positions, but are also able to improve on this by using pacing, improving their general aerobic fitness and strength, and paying more attention to body mechanics and posture.

Extended rest periods, or avoiding using the part of the body that is painful, are clearly detrimental. However, short regular and systematic rest periods are vital for the beneficial physiological effect on muscles and tissues. It also helps to prevent patterns of overactivity with subsequent muscle tension/spasm, as well as maximizing concentration and work performance. Many of us seem to have been brought up with the work ethic, feel guilty for taking breaks, have notions that it is bad to stop until a job is finished, and find it hard to say 'No' to others, always putting other people first. It is very rewarding to help patients discover that looking after themselves first actually helps them to deal more effectively and pleasantly with others. Equally, learning to delegate tasks, be assertive rather than submissive or aggressive, or to share tasks and do them together is also very rewarding for patients. It can feel very risky to take such new and big steps for some, though, so the smaller or more manageable the first step the better, until confidence has begun to build. This means that consequences such as fear or severe pain are minimized. Valued or pleasant consequences are also vital, as they help provide reinforcement for the activity and encourage its repetition despite pain (Harding 1998).

STRETCH

An unpublished audit undertaken at Guy's Hospital in 1986 asked patients with joint hypermobility what they found helpful, as there appeared to be little that physiotherapy could do. Very little emerged from this, except that several patients said they found stretch helpful. At the time this was a surprising finding for the authors, but subsequently this information, put together with further clinical experience, influenced the audit authors' approach to stretch. It was found that very gentle but sustained stretch proved to be a useful treatment and home exercise for pain and muscle spasm. However, many patients with joint hypermobility report that they have been previously told by health professionals: 'You've got "too much" movement', or 'You should never mobilize a hypermobile joint'. They have also been instilled with a fear of harm or damage, as they have been told that 'Pain equals damage', or this has been implied to them: 'You shouldn't do it if it hurts'; 'I wouldn't do it if I was you'; or 'Don't do *too* much'. Some have been told they should only do isometric exercise and no stretch, though one wonders if this is normal, or encourages normal relaxed movement.

Before it was discovered that so many patients attending INPUT had joint hypermobility the programme already contained an extensive stretch routine. Chronic pain patients frequently stiffen up from disuse, not only in their painful joints but, for many, in virtually all joints. The stretch routine aimed to cover practically all the active joint movements, and to stretch all the main muscle groups and mobilize major nerve trunks. Although this can only be described as anecdotal report, it is the impression that those with joint hypermobility can on the whole be separated from everyone else by their responses to the first stretch class. Even though strong and repeated emphasis is placed on doing the movements in an extremely gentle and very relaxed way, and not to go *through* pain, many patients look rather unhappy with the stretches; however, those with joint hypermobility seem to love it and are practically purring afterwards! It would seem reasonable to speculate that if hypermobile joints love stretching that much, they must be doubly uncomfortable if it is denied them. This denial can come as a result of the patients' own beliefs, but also from health professionals' bans on stretch.

MUSCLE SPASM AND TRIGGER POINTS

The literature does not seem to mention muscle spasm as a significant feature of hypermobility, but a combination of JHS and fibromyalgia has been reported (Goldman 1991, Gedalia et al. 1993, Hudson et al. 1995, Karaaslan et al. 2000, Holman and Fitzcharles 2002). Despite this lack of reference to muscle spasm in relation to hypermobility, the impression is that quite a few therapists have noted an increased tendency to muscle spasm in hypermobile patients. Clinical experience suggests that patients with joint hypermobility have many trigger points and areas of localized muscle spasm. These patients would often come in with a neck torticollis, an apparent sciatic scoliosis, or a quite severe limitation of range of any of their joints that responded extremely well to gentle joint mobilizations of the Maitland variety (Maitland 1986). The problem was that they would then return a day or two later with muscle spasm at another site. If treatment was continued in this way, the result was often chasing pain and muscle spasm all over the body. Teaching the patient self-management, using first aid, ice or warmth and very gentle sustained stretch, appeared to be much more successful. The suggestion is that patients with JHS can have more acute and flitting muscle spasm which can be more obvious than their milder chronic underlying muscle tension/chronic spasm, whereas the typical patient with fibromyalgia who does not have joint hypermobility has chronic muscle tension/spasm and muscle tightness as a major feature. It can be surmised that this may reflect underlying differences in their collagenous tissue properties, but as yet there is no way of confirming this.

Chronic pain management teaches patients with symptoms of muscle spasm and trigger points the self-help strategies described above, but in addition helps them to use effective relaxation and pacing to both prevent and ward off muscle spasm. An exploration of unhelpful thought patterns is also undertaken. These might include thoughts that encourage the person to push on with muscle tension, or make it hard to say 'No' to demands from other people that unwittingly undermine pacing. Thoughts or beliefs that sustain concerns about tissue fragility, rather than resilience, are addressed, as are worries about situations that tend to increase muscle tension and undermine confidence. It is surprising how well these patients can learn to manage situations themselves, how eventually they can break the muscle spasm cycle, and maintain longer spasm-free periods and overall reduced muscle tension.

Because some people with joint hypermobility also have many trigger points (Goldman 1991), it is worth learning from the trigger point/fibromyalgia literature. McCain (1986) and Goldman (1991), among others, have demonstrated the role of fitness training. Although the aetiology of fibromyalgia is barely understood, the protective effect of aerobic exercise is worth promoting, provided the hypermobile patient understands that it is doubly important for them to pace this up very gradually in order to prevent unmanageable pain flare-ups.

OTHERS' IMPRESSIONS OF JOINT HYPERMOBILITY

One would consider that people with joint hypermobility and pain have enough to cope with, yet their progress can sometimes be undermined by others. Sadly, this sometimes comes from inept remarks made by health professionals. Here is an extreme example:

Health professional: (Sharp intake of breath) 'I don't know how you manage to stand up/how your joints stay together/you must be constantly dislocating your joints, such a lot of damage'.

Even the public can contribute to this. A few patients report other people ridicule them or describe their movement as bendy and bizarre. Although some are commended for their graceful movement, it is suspected that abuse is more common than patients are willing to report.

Health professionals can certainly help here, so that rather than using words or phrases that indicate difference in a less than sympathetic way, they are complementary instead, e.g. 'You're wonderfully flexible/graceful, that's beautiful movement'. Better understanding from health professionals and society is certainly needed, and the work of self-help groups such as the Hypermobility Syndrome Association and the Ehlers–Danlos Support Group is very important here. Through education and publicity they are helping patients take control over how those with joint hypermobility are viewed and appreciated.

BEING DIFFERENT

It is very hard to live with chronic pain, but particularly when no-one can explain exactly what is wrong, or when you feel neglected or misunderstood. Many of our patients report that a valuable part of a pain management programme is meeting other patients with chronic pain, and hypermobility. For the first time they and their partners are relieved to realize that they are not the only person with chronic pain who doesn't get better, or have no explicable reason for their pain other than their hypermobility. Many have felt understandably mystified as to why they are different from others, and often felt quite isolated as a result. These feelings can help maintain a search for an answer or a cure, so a history of doctor, physiotherapist or alternative therapist 'shopping' is not uncommon. This in turn leads to swinging mood, with feelings of anticipatory excitement prior to more tests, trying new treatments or seeing a new specialist, followed by feelings of being let down by negative tests or treatment failure, and resultant depression (Pither and Nicholas 1991). As a result of treatment failure, some patients report having considered whether the pain might after all be 'in the mind', or even wondering about their own sanity. It is comforting to discover that others have shared their experience, and it is helpful to have an ex-patient return to talk to current patients about what it is like to manage chronic pain in the long term. Those who see hypermobile patients with pain for individual treatment can help by taking extra care to ensure they realize they are not unique, and that others with pain equally severe have, with persistent effort, had success in managing it themselves.

If no biomedical or mechanical cause for the patient's symptoms has been found, it can be easy for the patient to be labelled with a psychological or psychiatric cause. Evidence in the pain literature suggests that this is not the case and that a biopsychosocial model fits with the findings in patients (Main and Spanswick 2000). This means an acceptance that all pain has a biological cause, whether tissue damage or neurophysiological dysfunction, and that all patients with pain have a psychological response to it, as first proposed by the Gate Control Theory of Pain (Melzack and Wall 1965, Wall 1996). It is therefore important to reassure the patient that there is a biological basis for their pain and to challenge any thoughts they may have that there is a causative psychological factor. It is helpful to explain in simple terms the neurophysiological processes involved in chronic pain and, in addition, patients can be directed to very readable books on the subject, such as *The Challenge of Pain* (Melzack and Wall 1982) and *Pain: the Science of Suffering* (Wall 1999).

OPTIMIZING TREATMENT AND INCREASING PATIENT SATISFACTION

It is clear that useful information that relates to patients' own experiences and normalizes them is important. Information retention, however, is notoriously poor in any walk of life. This is particularly so when there are competing distractions such as pain operating, so good-quality handouts and written summaries of what has been said are important. Patients also appreciate:

- Practical tips – but again, write them down;
- The opportunity to try things out practically with good-quality feedback;

- To be taught skills;
- To gain a sense of control, often achieved by helping them explore their different options.

Patients are frequently grateful for the treatment they receive from health professionals. When treatment seems to help, though, it is worth investigating what it is that is helping. It is tempting for physiotherapists and doctors to think first of modalities and techniques that they have performed. When INPUT patients were asked about past treatment they mentioned the following factors as important:

- A sense of being believed ('they didn't think it was in my head/in my mind');
- 'Being listened to'
- The fact that someone cared. Some go on to qualify this: 'I don't mean being cared *for*, it's about being cared *about*';
- Good quality information:
  - 'It's MY problem, I need to know' (though it needs to be understandable);
  - 'I wasn't talked down to, patronized';
  - 'They gave me honest information, including "we don't know"';
  - 'I appreciated being credited with having a brain'.

It is remarkable how often patients say these sorts of things, rather than crediting the more technological or medical treatments. Patients report: 'I'd never have known I could do it unless I had tried and persevered', and some also report it saves them a lot of money in chiropractors' bills. Pain management will not make manipulative therapists redundant: they can still be very helpful for acute pain, and provided patients are prepared to take over responsibility and return to their self-help routine to keep pain and muscle spasm under control, they are a good support for when the patient is unable to fully manage a situation themselves. It does take skill, though, to recognize when a patient is using treatment rather than self-help, to elicit where the lack of confidence in self-management lies, then to help the person return to better long-term management rather than perpetuating ongoing crisis treatment that maintains dependency.

WHO CAN HELP HYPERMOBILE PATIENTS WITH THEIR CHRONIC PAIN MANAGEMENT?

With training and practice, most physiotherapists should be able to add cognitive–behavioural skills to their rehabilitation skills, thus enabling them to encourage self-management for lifetime conditions such as chronic pain (Harding 1998, Harding and Williams 1995). Increasingly, exercise groups are also utilizing cognitive–behavioural principles for pain conditions (Klaber Moffett et al. 1999). Unfortunately, there are still no published trials or descriptions of this approach used solely with JHS. The series of books *Topical Issues in Pain* produced by the Physiotherapy Pain Association, dealing admittedly with conditions other than JHS, give descriptions of how physiotherapists can use cognitive–behavioural pain management for their patients. Membership of the Physiotherapy Pain Association is available for a nominal subscription and its website can be found at: http://www.ppaonline.co.uk/. For hypermobile patients with more severe disability and distress due to chronic pain, it may be more appropriate to refer them on for an interdisciplinary chronic pain management programme. Generally patients who have at least two of the following due to their chronic pain are appropriate candidates:

- Widespread disruption in activity;
- Work reduced, impaired or ceased;
- Regular use of analgesics and/or sedatives without adequate relief;
- Clear signs/reports of emotional distress;
- Unnecessary use of aids (e.g. crutches, corset, wrist splints);
- High levels of pain behaviour.

A list of pain management programmes in the UK can be obtained from http://www.painsociety.org/sig_pain_man.htm.

CONCLUSION

There is circumstantial evidence to suggest that joint hypermobility is present in a higher proportion of the chronic pain population than might be expected, though not all these patients necessarily have JHS. Normal activity is still possible: it merely indicates that pacing up activity gradually, especially that involving strength or endurance, is more important for them. Anecdotally, stretch has been found to be helpful and should be balanced with activities that also strengthen and build endurance, using pacing.

Experience with chronic pain patients in a pain management setting suggests a number of possible markers for increased susceptibility and possible reasons for inadequate coping, though no firm evidence has yet emerged. However, chronic pain with joint hypermobility should perhaps be seen in the context of the neurophysiological mechanisms operating rather than as signs of tissue damage, and should encourage health professionals to take a biopsychosocial approach: explore beliefs, coping strategies, patterns of use and unhelpful habits that may have been taught or learnt.

Cognitive–behavioural pain management is successful in helping people with chronic pain and joint hypermobility improve and maintain their function, mood and joint health, and enables patients to accept that realizing that the pain will not necessarily go away is not an admission of failure.

The case study is of a patient who attended pain management in its early days in the UK. It is illustrative of some of the difficulties that chronic pain patients with joint hypermobility have, and how these can be overcome to the patient's satisfaction.

Case study

'Avoid stairs, never crouch, kneel or cycle, or you will get severe osteoarthritis by the time you are 40 from the chondromalacia due to your hypermobility.'

This comment was made to one of our hypermobile patients by her orthopaedic surgeon. She had been a nursing sister and her husband confirmed that this is what was said to them. She had already had a tensor fascia lata release operation for what was diagnosed as greater trochanteric bursitis following unaccustomed hill-walking. Consequently, when she and her husband first arrived at INPUT, he carried her piggy-back up the stairs to her room, ostensibly to prevent the osteoarthritis that they had been warned about. You can see in Table 10.1 the return to fitness and function that occurred when she was taught how to manage her pain. She had gained the confidence that exercise would reduce the chance of osteoarthritis later, and returned to climbing stairs, riding an exercise bicycle, squatting and kneeling, using a systematic pacing approach. At a pretreatment session she managed 17 stairs in 2 minutes, going up on her bottom. Her results 1 year after leaving the programme are impressive to say the least, and the fact that most improvement was made *after* finishing the 4-week programme demonstrates that teaching her self-management skills was what was most important. These are extracts from the letters she wrote to us:

'My walk is up to 17 minutes now, which means I can reach the local shops at last! It was a blow to realize I was not up to carrying while walking – having tried to buy up the greengrocer's in my elation at having got there for the first time! I restrict my shopping to 1 lb weight in each hand now, and that's OK.' (9 February 1990)

'Herewith the proceeds from a talk I gave about INPUT. I enjoyed our assessment day, although I was bushed afterwards: must have been the 210 stairs in 2 minutes! It occurred to me afterwards that the great thing is that it's no big deal. I know myself well enough now to make the adjustments accordingly and use a set-back plan if necessary.' (27 June 1990)

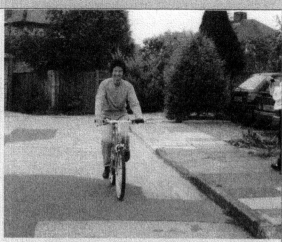

Figure 10.2 Case study: patient riding her bicycle

'I know you will be glad to hear I have bought a *real* bike at last! Very exciting – scary – and harder than I thought it would be, but I'm persevering and learning strictly INPUT-style!' (21 August 1990)

She sent a photograph of herself riding her bike (Fig. 10.2). (6 October 1990)

'I had a party to celebrate my first year of freedom. It was great fun, and the first party we had given for 6 years!' (18 January 1991)

She is now well over 40, has no signs of the predicted osteoarthritis she was dreading, and although she still has quite severe chronic pain, is able to cope with it. She has maintained her fitness and rates it generally greater now than when she was in her teens.

Table 10.1   Physical function test results before and after pain management

	Pre-treatment	Last day	1 month follow-up	6 month follow-up	1 year follow-up
10-minute walk (metres)	115	385	628	767	877
2-minute stand-ups	11	20	30	43	50
2-minute stair climb	17	38	78	210	229

REFERENCES

Acasuso, M., Collantes, E., Pujol, J. et al. (1994) Generalized articular hyperlaxity and musculoligamentous lesions. [Spanish] *Revista Española de Reumatologia*, **21**, 311–14.

Beighton, P.H, Solomon, L. and Soskolne, C.L. (1973) Articular mobility in an African population. *Annals of the Rheumatic Diseases*, **32**, 413–18.

Bulbena, A., Duro, J.C., Porta, M. et al. (1992) Clinical assessment of hypermobility of joints: assembling criteria. *Journal of Rheumatology*, **19**, 115–22.

Bulbena, A., Duro, J.C., Porta, M. et al. (1993) Anxiety disorders in the joint hypermobility syndrome. *Psychiatry Research*, **46**, 59–68.

Fairbank, J.C.T., Pynsent, P.B., van Poortvliet, J.A. and Phillips, H. (1984) Mechanical factors in the incidence of knee pain in adolescents and young adults. *Journal of Bone and Joint Surgery [British]*, **66B**, 685–93.

Flor, H., Fydrich, T. and Turk, D.C. (1992) Efficacy of multidisciplinary pain treatment centres: a meta-analytic review. *Pain*, **49**, 221–30.

Gedalia, A., Person, D.A., Brewer, E.J. Jr. and Giannini, E.H. (1985) Hypermobility of the joints in juvenile episodic arthritis/arthralgia. *Journal of Pediatrics*, **107**, 873–6.

Gedalia, A., Press, J., Klein, M. and Buskila, D. (1993) Joint hypermobility and fibromyalgia in schoolchildren. *Annals of the Rheumatic Diseases*, **52**, 494–6.

Goldman, J.A. (1991) Hypermobility and deconditioning: important links to fibromyalgia/fibrositis. *Southern Medical Journal*, **84**, 1192–6.

Grahame, R. (1999) Joint hypermobility and genetic collagen disorders. Are they related? *Archives of Disease in Childhood*, **80**, 188–91.

Grahame, R., Edwards, J.C., Pitcher, D. et al. (1981) A clinical and echocardiological study of patients with the hypermobility syndrome. *Annals of the Rheumatic Diseases*, **40**, 541–6.

Gratacos, M., Nadal, M. and Martin-Santos, R. (2001) A polymorphic genomic duplication on human chromosome 15 is a susceptibility factor for panic and phobic disorders. *Cell*, **106**, 367–79.

Harding, V.R. (1998) Application of the cognitive–behavioural approach. In: *Rehabilitation of Movement: Theoretical Basis of Clinical Practice* (J. Pitt-Brooke, ed). London: WB Saunders.

Harding, V.R. and Grahame, R. (1990) The frequency of joint hypermobility syndrome in chronic pain patients. *Pain*, **5** (Suppl), S500.

Harding, V.R. and Williams, A.C. de C. (1995) Extending physiotherapy skills using a psychological approach: managing chronic pain in a cognitive–behavioural multidisciplinary team. *Physiotherapy*, **81**, 681–8.

Holman, A.J. and Fitzcharles, M.-A. (2002) Is hypermobility a factor in fibromyalgia? [multiple letters]. *Journal of Rheumatology*, **29**, 396–8.

Hudson, N., Starr, M.R., Esdaile, J.M. and Fitzcharles, M-A. (1995) Diagnostic associations with hypermobility in rheumatology patients. *British Journal of Rheumatology*, **34**, 1157–61.

Karaaslan, Y., Haznedaroglu, S. and Öztürk, M. (2000) Joint hypermobility and primary fibromyalgia: a clinical enigma. *Journal of Rheumatology*, **27**, 774–6.

Klaber-Moffett, J., Torgerson, D., Bell-Syer, S. et al. (1999) Randomised controlled trial of exercise for low back pain: clinical outcomes, costs, and preferences. *British Medical Journal*, **319**, 279–83.

Main, C.J. and Spanswick, C.C. (2000) *Pain Management: An Interdisciplinary Approach*. Edinburgh: Churchill Livingstone.

Maitland, G.D. (1986) Principles of techniques. In *Vertebral Manipulation*, 5th edn. Butterworths.

McCain, G.A. (1986) Role of fitness training in the fibrositis/fibromyalgia syndrome. *American Journal of Medicine*, **81**, 73–7.

McNerny, J.E. and Johnston, W.B. (1979) Generalised ligamentous laxity, hallux abducto valgus and the first metatarsocuneiform joint. *Journal of the American Podiatric Association*, **69**, 69–82.

Melzack, R. and Wall, P.D. (1965) Pain mechanisms: a new theory. *Science*, **150**, 971–9.

Melzack, R. and Wall, P.D. (1982) *The Challenge of Pain*. Richard Clay, Chaucer Press Ltd, Suffolk.

Mikkelsson, M., Salminen, J. J. and Kautiainen, H. (1963) Joint hypermobility is not a contributing factor to musculoskeletal pain in pre-adolescents. *Journal of Rheumatology*, **23**, 1967.

Mishra, M.B., Ryan, P., Atkinson, P. et al. (1996) Extra-articular features of benign joint hypermobility syndrome. *British Journal of Rheumatology*, **35**, 861–6.

Morley, S., Eccleston, C. and Williams, A. (1999) Systematic review and meta-analysis of randomized controlled trials of cognitive behaviour therapy and behaviour therapy for chronic pain in adults, excluding headache. *Pain*, **80**, 1–13.

Pither, C.E. and Nicholas, M.K. (1991) The identification of iatrogenic factors in the development of chronic pain syndromes: abnormal treatment behaviour? In: *Proceedings of the VIth World Congress on Pain* (M.R. Bond, J.E. Charlton and C.J. Woolf, eds). Elsevier Science.

Spielberger, C.D. (1983) *Manual for the State–Trait Anxiety Inventory*. Paolo Alto, CA: Consulting Psychologists Press.

Wall, P.D. (1996) Comments after 30 years of the gate control theory. *Pain Forum*, **5**, 12–22.

Wall, P.D. (1999) *Pain: The Science of Suffering*. Phoenix.

Williams, A.C. de C. and Erskine, A. (1995) Chronic pain. In: *Health Psychology: Process and Applications*, 2nd edn. (A. Broome and S. Llewelyn, eds). London: Chapman & Hall.

11

Joint hypermobility syndrome from the patient's perspective

Sarah Gurley-Green

The Hypermobility Syndrome Association (HMSA) grew from the mutual frustration between patients and interested medical professionals about the poorly served needs of those suffering from this often disabling disorder. I served as chairperson for several years, often as a conduit between desperate patients and their doctors, trying to facilitate good communication. The HMSA began a number of years ago when a group of hypermobility syndrome patients from Guy's Hospital in London and medical practitioners with an interest in hypermobility were asked to attend a meeting to discuss participation in a support group for hypermobile patients. Around the conference table sat doctors, physiotherapists and patients. The patients were a good cross-section of the affected group in the general population. There were those who were very high functioning, many of whom were able to continue in full-time employment; there were those who were severely affected and dependent on disability benefits; many had sticks and canes, some had neck collars, arm braces, and a few had wheelchairs. What came across loud and clear was that some patients were very angry. Many had experienced poor treatment by the medical community in general, together with disbelief and lack of interest over a long period. They felt abandoned by the medical community, but at the same time wholly dependent upon it.

This group highlighted a problem prevalent within the medical system at large, particularly for the treatment of chronic pain: there exists a conflict of approach and perspective between the nature of the medical system and the patient;

it creates a power struggle, a conflict of authority. The patient requires help, and thus must give up some control. The system, and many of those practising in it, inclines toward the giving over of autonomy to the practitioner. Once that control is yielded, the lack of a successful outcome can have long-term effects on the patient's response to treatment in the future. The patient's need for answers is often not satisfied, and the patient may not be helped – perhaps may even be hurt – in the process of treatment. Over many years patients become angry and powerless, disillusioned and impotent to help themselves, and difficult and frustrating to treat.

In the process of running the HMSA several issues became clear. First, there is poor communication and a lack of understanding between patients and the medical community. Second, joint hypermobility syndrome (JHS) is difficult to diagnose, underdiagnosed, and often diagnosed late in the patient's experience with the disorder. Third, JHS is difficult both for medical practitioners to treat and for patients to control and to effect any meaningful change upon their condition.

Broadly, JHS patients fall into two groups. Some are more mildly affected and suffer periodic injuries and pain; after effective treatment they can resume normal lives. However, there is a significant minority who are more severely affected and whose lives are a daily struggle with injury and pain. Risk of injury (anticipated or unexpected), probable pain and tiredness are all baggage that must be carried by many on every journey. These activities can be as mundane as caring for one's personal needs of dressing and bathing, shopping, or any repetitive movement such as chopping, walking, lifting and carrying. There are many consequences of chronic pain and fear of pain – physical, psychological and social. The majority of the members of the HMSA fall into this more affected group. The Association has grown over the last several years. It now has a website (www.hypermobility.org), newsletters, international support groups, and successful informational residential weekends. All are testament to the tenacity of its members. The strength of need is shown by the over 25 000 hits per week to the website.

There are significant difficulties in the diagnosis and treatment of all hypermobile patients. For the physiotherapist, in the diagnosis of injury and subsequent treatment special consideration must be given to the large range of movement found in these patients. Reported stiffness and perceived abnormalities of (passive) movement are not effective as diagnostic tools in assessing a hypermobile patient for four reasons:

1. These patients may appear to have better than average range of movement even when there is an injury.
2. The excessive flexibility of another area can compensate for a lack of movement in the affected or injured part.
3. Patients may report stiffness that does not appear to agree with examination.
4. For many patients stiffness and pain are overlapping concepts: reported stiffness may mean loss of movement due to pain to the patient. The reported stiffness may not be apparent to an observer on examination, as the range of movement looks normal.

A further problem in assessing these patients is that their explanation of an event or accident may not equate to the degree of injury or pain suffered. The patient may not even recall any event that may have caused the pain. The reason for this may be that only everyday activities were involved, such as shopping, making the beds or making dinner, but also because the pain often takes several hours or even days to appear. Everyday activities can be a cause of pain, swelling and subluxation, which in another patient would have required severe trauma to effect such an injury. This is a good diagnostic signal to a switched-on practitioner, but may have also been a source of less-aware practitioners determining that the pain was psychosomatic or the injury self-inflicted.

Typically, JHS patients have had symptoms since childhood or early adolescence; most patients had their first symptom by the age of 20. Their flexibility may have been thought of as an asset: it may have encouraged them to dance or perform gymnastics. They might always have experienced pain afterwards, but they managed to get through it until such time as an acute episode or injury forced them to seek professional help, and eventual diagnosis. Others may not have been strong enough for such physical activities and may have been thought of as lazy or somewhat hypochondriacal. The patient might have never been able to tell the doctor what had caused the pain, and therefore their veracity was doubted. In most cases the pain and the doubt have gone on for years before eventual diagnosis. This typical history of hypermobile patients makes communicating with a doctor difficult. As a result, and in common with many chronic pain syndromes, most JHS patients and their families view medical professionals with scepticism.

Years of suffering pain and disability can cause loss of status within the society in which they live as the illness forces them to terminate their careers, fractures family relationships and narrows their world through social isolation. Even after the correct diagnosis has been made (which, in itself, may give a temporary sense of wellbeing) the generally available conventional treatment is, on the whole, ineffective. For the majority of patients the first symptom is pain. It is the symptom that causes the most disruption to daily life for JHS sufferers.

Although swelling and obvious dislocations of joints are not uncommon for hypermobile patients, the most commonly reported symptom is pain. This fact alone makes successful assessment and treatment difficult. Primarily, pain is a subjective symptom: its only true measurement is the patient's own reporting. According to the National Academy of Sciences Institute of Medicine's report on Pain and Disability, there is no thermometer for pain, no absolutely reliable quantitative, independent method of evaluating the severity or frequency of the symptom in individual subjects (Osterweis et al. 1987).

The medical practitioner must rely on the patient's ability to report pain accurately in order to treat it effectively. It is most important, then, that communication be effective and open, doubly so to combat the commonplace feeling of patients that they are burdensome and in some way responsible for their condition.

The vocabulary of pain is imprecise, leaving the patient isolated by their inability to articulate the impact of pain and dominated by its all-consuming nature. Like a fire that takes on a life of its own, for many patients pain is a force that is at times overwhelming. Visual Analogue Pain Scales from 1 to 10 are in widespread use in clinical research, but they cannot express the suffering accurately. It is common to hear a chronic pain patient report that their pain is a '12 out of 10' (Good et al. 1992a). Such a statement expresses the frustration a person in severe pain feels at their inability to communicate their suffering and their fear about its uncontrollability. Doctors and physiotherapists may suspect that this amplification is due to psychological problems, without appreciating that it is symptomatic of the patient's inability to express the crushing effect of their pain. This can lead to frustration and misunderstanding, potentially creating or exacerbating a climate of mistrust.

Many people with hypermobility are in daily pain. As with other chronic pain disorders, the patient's response to noxious stimuli may be altered and sensitized through long-term pain and inflammation. For many medical practitioners the understanding of pain is dominated by the idea that injury means pain and pain means injury, and that there is a causal and connecting line between the two. A medical practitioner will often ask the patient, 'What have you done?' The hypermobile patient may not know; moreover, the very nature of the question may appear accusatory. Sensitization over many years causes some hypermobile patients to report that even being touched can cause pain. This hyperalgesia or allodynia can be troubling to sufferers and their families, particularly when there has been a history of disbelief by the medical community.

Pain has more than a quantitative element: it has a qualitative one as well. The description and particular characterization of different pains makes it problematic to report accurately or evaluate. For example, hypermobile patients often complain of 'stiffness', but what they feel has no relation to the common definition of stiffness that may be experienced by anyone with arthritis, or a healthy person who overexerts himself. Moreover, when he or she reports to the physiotherapist that they are stiff, unlike a patient with arthritis, upon examination they will be highly mobile.

In JHS fear of pain is often as debilitating as the pain itself. This is because the pain is both chronic and acute. This fear both prevents compliance with self-managed exercise regimens given by the doctor and physiotherapist and causes isolation from the world, affecting social relationships and the pursuance of life goals. When a hypermobile person exercises he or she is in pain afterwards. We have found anecdotally that those JHS patients who do exercise regularly reduce chronic pain in the long term, and also reduce the number of acute pain episodes and injuries such as subluxations. However, it requires enormous willpower and self-efficacy for an individual to do something he or she knows will cause them pain in the short term. There is a strong relationship between the severity of painful symptoms and poor self-efficacy for exercise (Barlow 1988). On the other hand, a number of sufferers have stated that the quality of pain after exercise is often less severe than that from an acute episode. This highlights the importance of patients trying to describe their pain in qualitative terms, and also the need for a more precise means of communicating this in response to treatment and exercise programmes. Non-compliance in a JHS patient may not mean they are ignoring the doctor's advice, but rather that they are actually listening to their body's direction and instruction.

Cognitive–behavioural treatment methods may be effective as part of pain management, but it may require special consideration for the patient who has suffered a long history of disbelief and lack of interest from the medical community. For a hypermobile person in chronic pain, every aspect of work and family life has been altered by this disorder. Often, a hypermobile patient would have had to plead a case for the legitimacy of his or her pain before a sceptical physician. The hypermobile patient looks well and may have a large range of movement while complaining of severe pain, and must campaign for the validity and physicality of the pain. In some cases the vulnerability of the patient's self-esteem and relations with the world may be tied to the concept that pain has no psychological or subjective element, and he or she can appear resistant to cognitive behavioural methods initially. In addition, asked how an injury occurred or what triggered the pain, many JHS patients will be unable to trace to a specific event. This may be due either to sensitization through long-standing pain and inflammation, or injury due to everyday activities, such as lifting, walking, shopping, etc. Therefore, behaviour modification is difficult if one does not know precisely what behaviour caused the injury in the first place.

Research supports the view that self-help and patient-led management is currently the best long-term approach for the treatment of JHS. This can be problematic for JHS patients, for several reasons:

- The syndrome robs the patient of control and order.
- The seemingly random nature of the disorder means that one is unable to know whether one will be well, or in bed in severe pain.
- The ability to plan and order one's life is denied.
- Chronic pain causes feelings of loss of control, depression and inertia. This makes a belief in one's ability to effect positive change in one's life difficult.
- In addition, the fear of pain can be paralysing, as patients do not have a clear understanding of their pain and the cause and effect relationship between an event and subsequent pain.

- An unclear understanding of their bodies' limits may cause poor self-esteem and body awareness. This may result in a down-spiralling of patients' strength through progressive physical inactivity.

JHS has an impact upon the psychosocial functioning of the sufferer, including problems with self-management. The body in which we live influences our understanding of who we are and where we fit into the society in which we live, or our self-concept. JHS can profoundly influence a patient's self-concept and how that patient then is able to cope with symptoms. In chronic illness suffering is an ever-present state from which the patient cannot distance himself, and he may internalize negative definitions of self: ' ... the disruption of the taken-for-granted world of everyday life ... caused by chronic illness can be seen as nothing less than an ontological assault affecting the concept of self and not merely the performance of activities' (Good et al. 1992b).

Successful self-management requires the patient to have an internal sense of control, to feel that he or she can change life for the better by changing their behaviour. This self-empowerment is difficult if the patient has a long history of seeking many types of treatment, seeing many medical practitioners and scores of physical therapists, resulting in a lack of continuity, disbelief and conflicting advice, thereby making the patient feel more helpless and less empowered. It is vital for the successful treatment of this chronic problem for the patient to feel empowered, in touch with his or her internal locus of control, and to feel like a partner in the treatment. Patient involvement with the Hypermobility Syndrome Association support group has shown that identification with other patients and education about the disorder can have a very positive and empowering effect. Ultimately, however, it is difficult for the physical therapist to express a need for the patient to take responsibility for his treatment and recovery without implying that he is responsible or accountable for the pain. The patient

needs to feel responsible for his health in the sense that he has the self-efficacy that is necessary for successful self-management. However, the patient may feel capable of controlling his or her illness when control may not in fact be a realistic goal. The patient needs to differentiate between aspects of the illness that can be altered and those that cannot. 'Making this differentiation decreases distress by providing suitable targets for coping; inability to make the differentiation can result in failure, loss of control, and increased emotional distress caused by efforts to change the unchangeable' (Contrada and Ashmore 1999).

The patient needs to learn to struggle *with* their illness, not against it (Charmaz 1995). When he struggles *against* it the patient retains hope of regaining his past identity after vanquishing the enemy of the illness. He continues to loathe himself as well as the illness. On the contrary, when he struggles *with* the illness there is a shift to accepting the body's limitations while exploring what it can still do. In this process, the patient learns to protect the body and to extend it, thereby gaining control over the illness. Greater belief in the ability to control the illness leads to greater self-efficacy and hence better compliance with self-managed exercise programmes and pacing of activities.

In 1994, a multidisciplinary study of Ehlers–Danlos syndrome (EDS) conducted in the USA found that significantly higher levels of psychosocial problems occurred in type III EDS and joint hypermobility syndrome patients than in those with types I and II EDS. The authors state: 'The severe joint problems in EDS type III and the clinically similar JHS appear to lead to chronic, often debilitating pain which may explain the increased psychosocial disturbances reported by these patients' (Lumley et al. 1994). When comparing psychiatric symptoms and pain the differences between EDS type III/JHS and types I/II EDS shows significant difference for depression, anxiety, total numbers of psychiatric symptoms, and pain severity and interference in daily life. This American sample showed that 71% had received some psychiatric services at some point in their lives. In the interview process, however, they reported being disturbed by the psychiatric referral process and the reactions of mental health professionals. For many who have fought against disbelief and suspicion from the medical community, any question of psychological involvement seems to threaten the validity of their suffering. The question of responsibility for their pain vs. responsibility for their health may make the patient feel the psychiatric community is attributing blame (Good et al. 1992c). The high levels of depression and anxiety alone should make the use of mental health practitioners a useful tool to these patients.

Patients should be encouraged to keep a narrative of their illness, not merely to identify which activity exacerbates the symptoms, but as a heuristic understanding of the experience of the illness. In addition, it can be a tool for the medical professional to make and update a plan of treatment and to base advice on the patient's individual experience (Contrada and Ashmore 1999). There is still poor communication in what are often strained relationships between medical practitioner and JHS patient.

Patients who use support groups are often doing so as a result of dissatisfaction with the medical community. Reading the comments and views on the www.hypermobility.org website one gains a perspective that the members are using the support group to differentiate between symptoms and self, to validate suffering, and to seek community and unconditional understanding of their suffering. Its usefulness, though, goes far beyond these factors, not least as a means of identifying the complex issues broached in this chapter. It has already started to provide a forum for a more methodical appreciation of what JHS is, in particular its complexity and diversity among individual sufferers, and to evaluate what does and does not provide help to them. The patients must be active partners in the planning and management of their treatment. This will give them empowerment and self-efficacy. JHS is a lifelong disorder filled with pain and often unwanted medical involvement. Good communication with the patient as partner is paramount because self-management, with good physical therapy for acute episodes, may be the only long-term option for effective treatment.

REFERENCES

Barlow, J.H. (1988) Understanding exercise in the context of chronic disease: an exploratory investigation of self efficacy. *Perceptual and Motor Skills*, **87**, 444.

Charmaz, K. (1995) The body, identity and self: adapting to impairment. *Sociological Quarterly*, **36**, 671.

Contrada, R.J. and Ashmore, R.D. (1999) *Self, Social Identity and Physical Health*. Oxford University Press.

Good, M-J.D., Brodwin, P.E., Good, B.J. and Kleinman, A. (1992a) *Pain as Human Experience: An Anthropological Perspective*, pp. 181. University of California Press.

Good, M-J.D., Brodwin, P.E., Good, B.J. and Kleinman, A. (1992b) *Pain as Human Experience:*

An Anthropological Perspective, pp. 104. University of California Press.

Good, M.-J.D., Brodwin, P.E., Good, B.J. and Kleinman, A. (1992c) *Pain as Human Experience: An Anthropological Perspective*, pp. 160. University of California Press.

Lumley, M.A., Jordan, M., Rubinstein, R. et al. (1994) Psychosocial functioning in the Ehlers–Danlos syndrome. *American Journal of Medical Genetics*, **53**, 149–52.

Osterweis, M., Kleinman, A., Mechanic, D. (eds) (1987) *Pain and Disability: Clinical, Behavioral and Public Policy Perspectives*, p 3–4. Washington DC: National Academy Press.

Index

Printed and bound by CPI Group (UK) Ltd, Croydon, CR0 4YY

03/10/2024

01040345-0015